Outreach with the Elderly

Clinical Gerontology
GENERAL EDITOR: *Steven H. Zarit*

OUTREACH
WITH THE ELDERLY
Community Education, Assessment, and Therapy

Bob G. Knight

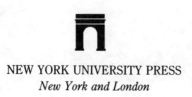

NEW YORK UNIVERSITY PRESS
New York and London

Library of Congress Cataloging-in-Publication Data

Knight, Bob.
    Outreach with the elderly : community education, assessment, and
therapy / Bob G. Knight.
        p.   cm. — (Clinical gerontology ; 2)
    Bibliography: p.
    Includes index.
    ISBN 0-8147-4597-0
    1. Aged—Mental health services, 2. Community mental health
services I. Title. II. Series.
    [DNLM: 1. Community Mental Health Services—in old age—United
States. 2. Home Care Services. 3. Psychotherapy—in old age.
4. Psychotherapy—methods.   WT 30 K690]
RC451.4.A5K587   1989
362.2′084′6—dc20
DNLM/DLC
for Library of Congress   89-9409
                                                                                        CIP

New York University Press books are printed on acid-free paper,
and their binding materials are chosen for strength and durability.

Contents

Acknowledgments

The program described in this book gradually grew as a truly interactive team effort within a community of service providers who shaped its focus and efforts and within a historical context of planning and development by the Ventura County Mental Health Department. During the years described here, first William Keating, M.D., and then Jack Graham, L.C.S.W., were the directors of that department. The training efforts for staff described in chapter 2 were under the direction of Andrew McCashin, Ph.D. The community services efforts and especially the Creative Aging Workshops were under the direction of Richard Reinhart, Ph.D.

Full-time members of the Senior Outreach Team through the period described in this book included Barbara Peterson Roth, R.N., L.C.S.W., and Marianne Slaughter, L.C.S.W., who comprised the original team and contributed substantially to the development of the outreach, assessment, and therapy components. Barbara Roth has since become the program manager of the team. Patricia Field, M.D., was the team psychiatrist from 1981 to 1988 and was instrumental in developing health assessments and the appropriate use of psychotropic medication, in improving our relationship with the medical community, and in increasing the team's concern for the schizophrenic and paranoid elderly. Adela Browne, R.N., G.N.P., provided the outreach to the Hispanic elderly and also served as an effective advocate for the older severely mentally ill clients. Barbara Kurtz, R.N., and Scott Jones, M.S.G., L.C.S.W., joined the team in later years and helped to deepen and refine the assessment and psychotherapeutic services. Sam Gotlieb, L.C.S.W., was with the team briefly before his death in 1987 and deserves special mention for his sharing of insights into the differences between working with the elderly and other age groups and the emotional impact of work with older adults. Virginia Hedman was our clerical staff from the beginning until her retirement in 1988 and assisted in a million ways with office procedures, organizational development, and tracking data.

The team's thinking about dementia and development of services for the demented elderly and their families was extensively influenced by the University of Southern California's Andrus Older Adult Center, then directed by Steven Zarit, Ph.D., and Nancy Orr, M.S.G., The first caregivers we worked with also shaped our thinking. Chapter 6 also benefitted from my discussion with other members of the California Alzheimer's Disease Task Force and the testimony of dozens of people at our public hearings.

Extensive interaction with elderly clients and with the community of older residents of Ventura County, California, has contributed greatly to the development of the program and of this book. Their appreciation of our successes and candid criticism of our failures have been a principal source of learning for me.

As the series editor, Steven Zarit, Ph.D., is responsible for the idea of this book and has guided me throughout the writing of it. Kitty Moore at New York University Press has been helpful and enthusiastic in facilitating its publication. Margaret Cortese, Ph.D., has been most helpful in shaping my ideas about outreach to Hispanics and the process of outreach more generally in countless conversations over ten years. She also loaned me her computer to complete the typescript when I suddenly found myself without one.

Margaret Gatz, Ph.D., and Cynthia Pearson, Ph.D., both of the University of Southern California, and Sandra Powers, Ed.D., of the University of North Carolina at Greensboro, have each been instrumental in shaping my thinking about the outreach team. They helped me to see unusual aspects of the team that I had grown to take for granted.

Chapter 8 appeared in a slightly different form in the *International Journal of Aging and Human Development* (copyright 1986, Baywood Publishing) as two articles: "Therapists' attitudes as an explanation of underservice to the elderly in mental health: Testing an old hypothesis," 22 *IJAHD* (1986) 261–69 and "Management variables as predictors of service utilization by the elderly in mental health," 23 *IJAHD* (1986) 141–48.

Part of chapter 9 is adapted from "Assessing a mobile outreach team" which appeared as a chapter in M. A. Smyer and M. Gatz, eds., *Mental health and aging: Programs and evaluations.* Beverly Hills: Sage, 1983. Copyright Sage Publications, 1983.

Chapter 11 includes material published as: "Factors influencing therapist-rated change in older adults," *Journal of Gerontology* 43 (1988) 11–12. Copyright 1988 by the Gerontological Society of America.

Part I
THE MODEL PROGRAM

1

The Elderly and Mental Health Services

Most older Americans have little contact with the mental health system. This has become an increasing focus of public interest in the 1980s. The public mental health sector now recognizes the elderly as a special population, and the aging services and planning sectors realize that older people have a need for mental health services. Older people have increasingly been seen as a special population to be served by mental health centers, and successive revisions of the Older Americans' Act have emphasized the need to include mental health services in that system of care. There is every indication that these policy changes will continue and perhaps even increase in the next decade and into the next century as the proportion of older citizens continues to grow.

The recognition of need has grown but the understanding of the problem has not deepened. Most discussions of mental health and aging focus on the lack of services and merely express the hope that someone will do something. There is still a persistent tendency to assume that all elderly, or at least most needing mental health care, suffer from brain impairments, such as Alzheimer's disease, and are therefore untreatable. Classifying the elderly as a "special population" assumes that the system is biased against them. Attempts to correct this bias by emphasizing normal aging have sometimes obscured the real needs of those elderly who suffer from psychiatric disorders. It is clear that the relationship between the mental health system and both academic gerontology and the aging services network has not been well developed or well planned (Knight 1986a; Fleming et al. 1986).

OVERVIEW OF THIS BOOK

Our conceptual analysis of the low rates of use of community-based mental health services by older adults is built on four points. First, recent data on prevalence rates of mental disorder in late life and on service utilization across the adult life span suggest that the problem may be less severe and less specific to the elderly than previously thought. There are also indications that the rate of the use of services by the elderly has been increasing. Second, a review of barriers to outpatient mental health services for older adults and how to overcome them provided us with specific direction as to how to reach the elderly population. Third, an analysis of types of frailty among the elderly clarifies the potential role of mental health treatment in prolonging home-based care for this group. Finally, a description of the range of institutional and home-based care for older adults shows the context within which the mental health geriatric specialist will operate.

This conceptual analysis, described in this chapter, led us to pursue a number of different strategies for the development of an outreach team. First, we stressed the need for education about mental health for older people and aging services providers and for training about aging for mental health providers. Second we used sliding scale fees and home-delivered services to overcome economic and physical barriers. Third, the services themselves emphasized the need for accurate and thorough assessments to guide active treatment interventions for those elderly who could benefit from outpatient services.

The development of the outreach team is described in chapter 2 while the specific services are described in chapters 3 through 5. Chapter 6 focuses on mental health interventions for the demented elderly and their families. Chapter 7 discusses some of the emotional hazards of work with this population for mental health team members, an important consideration in training and in maintaining staff morale. The team described here also used clinical research and program evaluation to enhance understanding of client needs and the outreach process and to monitor the effectiveness of its efforts. This research program is described in the second section of this book, in chapters 8 through 11.

There are certain questions one should ask in discussing the relationship of the elderly and the mental health system. How many of the elderly need mental health services? Do they underutilize mental health services in comparison to their need, and if so, why? Does our experience with other populations and with the elderly themselves suggest ways to improve rates of service use? Which elderly can mental health services help and how? How can mental health services fit into the larger system of care for older adults?

UTILIZATION AND THE NEED FOR MENTAL HEALTH SERVICES

It is widely known that the elderly underutilize outpatient mental health services relative to their representation in the population. In 1983 the elderly comprised 11% of the population and 6% of users of community mental health (Fleming et al. 1986), with lower representation in other clinics and still lower in private practices. In recent years, more of the elderly have begun to use mental health services. In the early 1970s, 4% of those who used community mental health centers were elderly (see Butler and Lewis 1977; Redick and Taube 1980; Gatz et al. 1985). By 1983, this figure had risen to 6% (Fleming et al. 1986). Redick and Taube (1980) note that this is not due to an increase in the population of elderly alone in that the use of community mental health rose from 72.9 per 100,000 to 164.8 per 100,000 and for all outpatient services from 101.0 per 100,000 to 237.0 per 100,000 in the 1971 to 1975 period. Without major new program initiatives, things have changed for the better. Unfortunately, we do not have studies that can suggest why.

Early reports from the National Institute of Mental Health (NIMH) Catchment Area Survey (a national research program to assess the need for and use of mental health services by all age groups) give reason to question whether the target of representation by percentage of population is appropriate for the elderly. These studies suggest that aside from cognitive impairment and phobia, six-month prevalence rates of mental disorder decrease in older age groups. Persons under 45 appear to have about twice as much psychiatric disorder as persons over 45 (Myers and Associates 1984). The same series of studies indicates an interesting anomaly in the lifetime prevalence rates for mental disorder: while we would logically expect lifetime prevalence rates for most psychiatric disorders to increase in the successively older groups of subjects, this increase was observed only for cognitive impairment. As the authors note, this finding raises such questions as: Do older people have differential mortality, out-migration, or institutionalization patterns? Are they likely to forget symptoms or to attribute symptoms to physical illness? Or has there been a true historical increase in mental disorder within the last few generations? (Robins and Associates 1984). Yet another problem may lie in reliance on the Folstein Mini-Mental Status exam for diagnosis of cognitive impairment; Folstein, Folstein, and McHugh (1975) themselves note that the scale picks up cognitive impairment due to psychiatric disorders as well as to dementing illness. It is unclear in these reports whether the authors were sensitive to the possibility of cognitive impairment being due to other than organic brain syndrome disorders. Less educated older people may also test impaired on the Folstein even when they are not in fact cognitively impaired by reason of dementia or psychiatric disorder (Folstein et al. 1985).

The diagnosis of mental disorder in the elderly is generally problematic; therefore, epidemiological studies and estimates are hard to interpret. Ranges for depression in older adults vary dramatically; some argue that rates are under 2% to others higher than 20% (Romanuik, McAuley, and

Arling 1983; Blazer, Hughes, and George 1987). While much hinges on how one, draws the line between sadness or low life satisfaction and clinical depression (Blazer, Hughes, and George argue, for example, that about 19% are "dysphoric" whereas 8% had a depressive diagnosis or symptoms), LaRue, Dessonville, and Jarvik (1985) note that the interviewers' diagnostic style may explain most of the variance in reported rates of mental disorder in older people.

These findings raise important issues. The elderly, while underserved at present, may be relatively more healthy and not require as much service as population rates might suggest. This question is far from settled, but we need a more sophisticated analysis than population equity. The population equity argument also obscures possible group differences such as the importance of cognitive impairment and phobias in the older population as suggested by the NIMH/Catchment-area Epidemiological Survey (CES) studies cited above.

The utilization studies from that project provide yet another perspective on the low use of services by the aged. The utilization rates of mental health services varied both in terms of the three sites and in terms of older and younger clients. Also, this report points out the discrepancy between need and use. For all adults, only 15% to 20% of those with mental disorders sought help, with only 8% to 12% visiting a mental health specialist. On the other hand, about 33% of persons with mental health visits had no mental disorder. While the elderly had a low utilization rate, their rate was not lower than that of the youngest group of adults, 18–24 years of age (Shapiro and Associates 1984). Clearly, more study is required to determine the need for services, the problem of low utilization of services may need to be conceptualized as similar to problems in other target populations, and our arguments should be more complex than simply saying, "There aren't many elderly here. There should be more."

Second, the increased number of cognitively impaired elderly, many of whom suffer from irreversible brain impairment, poses the dilemma of whether they should be categorized as mental health clients. This decision is likely to vary state by state, as does the decision to use separate service systems for the developmentally disabled and substance abusers. The decision will have an impact on the type and scope of programming for the elderly. Given their different needs, the two groups will use different types of services. It is of critical importance not to confuse the two and especially not to assume that an elderly person will be cognitively impaired. In addition, with the brain-impaired older person, as with others who are severely disabled, the caregiver may be in need of mental health services to be able to provide in-home care.

BARRIERS TO SERVICES FOR THE ELDERLY

Many reasons have been advanced for the low use of mental health services among the elderly. Several authors have argued that age discrimination makes mental health therapists prejudiced against (Butler and Lewis 1977) or afraid of older clients (Kastenbaum 1964). Others have pointed out the stigma against mental health care and have argued that the elderly have misconceptions and an active prejudice against mental health services (Patterson 1976; General Accounting Office 1982). There is also lack of training or information for therapists. I have argued that therapists may feel that working with the elderly demands special expertise and skills and that for this reason they avoid such work because they feel incompetent in this area (1986a, 1986b). Moreover, some elderly may simply not see their problems as psychological, or they may be unaware of the existence of outpatient therapy. Furthermore, services for older people may not be physically accessible to them. Availability of transportation, use of home visits, handicap accessibility, and location in acceptable surroundings are all issues that must be considered in providing services to the elderly.

Finally, it must be recognized that many elderly are either poor or feel that they should save their funds for future health crises (Butler and Lewis 1977; Knight 1986a). Cost of services is thus most certainly a factor in the elderly's differential use of community mental health clinics versus private practice.

POTENTIAL SOLUTIONS TO THESE BARRIERS

Most discussions of the problem of barriers to services for the elderly end with a list of specific issues. I will go one step further and consider solutions to these problems. First, if therapists are, in fact, prejudiced against the elderly, what can be done about it? One study I conducted showed that this prejudice was not present in a sample of therapists surveyed, but there is no doubt a range of feelings against the elderly (1986b). Any system that handles a variety of different client groups is aware that not all therapists can work with any one population. The elderly are not the only group against whom therapists may have prejudices. Some may feel incapable of working with the developmentally disabled, the long-term mentally ill, physically disabled persons, minority group members, or children. Rather than perceiving age-prejudice as a pervasive influence, bias against the elderly, in this view, is seen as a characteristic of some therapists. It then becomes a management issue to be considered in hiring therapists for an age-specific program or in assigning cases within an age-integrated program.

Second, what can be done about the obstensible stigma against mental health? This stigma is often presented as a pervasive and insurmountable barrier; experience, however, has shown it to be neither of those. A long history of case reports (Rechtschaffen 1959; Knight 1978–1979, 1986a, 1986b) has shown at least some elderly to be receptive to therapy and to benefit from it. Clearly there are people in all age groups who are very biased against mental health services and who will refuse them. The two large-scale studies available to date argue that this bias does not increase with age. Once a problem is seen as psychological in nature, the old are as likely to seek professional help as the young (Gurin, Veroff, and Feld 1960; Veroff, Koulka, and Douvan 1981).

Third, it may be that both therapists and potential older clients do not have enough information about each other. Therapists certainly need to have specific assessment skills and working knowledge of the existing network of services for the aged. They also need to feel comfortable in dealing with the issues that tend to arise in this group (including disability, illness, death) and to understand the nature of the aging experience. Potential clients may need help in recognizing their problems as psychological and in understanding the process of therapy and how it may help with their problem. This lack of information on both sides can be remedied by education. Therapists need additional training, continuing education, and inservice programs. The elderly need clear explanations of the process and benefits of mental health intervention and an understanding of the types of services available to them, both of which can be addressed through community education.

Fourth, the issue of accessibility of services, long a cornerstone of the community mental health movement (Little 1976), is critical for a population with limited ability to get around. The aged need a facility close to public transportation, accessible to handicapped persons, and located in a safe neighborhood in which they feel at home. For those unable to come to the clinic, home visits are crucial. In many communities, the elderly may need an office in a location away from programs serving younger mentally ill or substance abusing clients and away from the psychiatric hospital, quite often a key element in the fears of older people.

Fifth, the cost of private mental health care may make this service out of reach to most elderly. Whether they simply lack the money or want to keep their savings to finance future health care, many elderly are unable or unwilling to pay full private practice rates for mental health services. Yet most who need such services are willing to pay something. Any attempt to fully meet the need of this population will depend on finding a mix of outside funding and a sliding fee scale to make this service affordable. This formula will depend on expanding Medicare and Medicaid funding (both of which are much more generous for inpatient care at this point), inclusion of mental health benefits in private insurance, and the willingness of providers to use a reasonable system of sliding fees.

The focus so far has been on the underuse of outpatient services by older persons with no prior contact with the mental health system. There is another group for whom mental health services are critical: those elderly who had received institutional care from the mental health system in the past and continue to need services. The following discussion directs attention to the existence of this group: the long-term mentally ill who grow old.

DEINSTITUTIONALIZATION AND THE ELDERLY

As was true for most age groups, mental health services for the elderly prior to 1955 were mainly delivered by the state hospital system and consisted of long-term confinement in large institutional environments. Since few patients of any age were expected to improve, programs were often organized by age rather than by diagnosis. There was relatively little concern with distinguishing between residents who had been mentally ill for life and those who had become mentally ill late in life. With the advent of psychotropic medications and the move toward local mental health programming, most elderly were moved from the state hospital system to nursing homes and residential care homes (Kahn 1977; Redick and Taube 1980; General Accounting Office 1982; Shadish 1983, 1984). Some argue that the younger chronically mentally ill suffered a similar fate in what is usually described euphemistically as "returning patients to the community" (Shadish 1983, 1984) and might more realistically be seen as a move from large, state-financed institutions to smaller, more locally based, privately and federally financed institutions (Rounds 1982).

Many have argued that the promise to provide community-based services was not kept for any age group. Certainly this was the case for the elderly client. The older mental patient went from infrequent contact with psychiatry to no contact at all (Kahn 1977; General Accounting Office 1982). In fact, in the new environment of the long-term medical care system, the clients were labelled either as physically ill or as simply old. Attention to mental disorders such as schizophrenia and depression has been minimal in these settings, and the understanding of organic disorders such as Alzheimer's disease and multi-infarct dementia is often obscured by the perception of the effects of these processes as normal aging. This misperception has both deprived these patients of needed specialized care and exposed those patients who are in nursing homes for convalescence after heart surgery or other physical illness to an odd social environment and a depressing vision of their own aging. And for the mentally ill elderly, the long-term care facilities are inadequate for their needs. Skilled nursing facilities are intended to provide convalescent care after acute medical hospital admission. Residential care homes are intended for the nonspecific problems of aging. The elderly psychiatric patient is left as a square peg in a round hole in either setting. The cognitively impaired patient, probably the majority of residents in both types of long-term care for the elderly, has no intentionally designed program at all.

As we have seen, even as the most severe cases were moved from one institution to another, the less severely impaired elderly have tended to be neglected altogether by community-based mental health programming. Consciously or otherwise, community mental health programs have tended to operate on the philosophy that their services are most appropriate for the younger person with mental or emotional distress and to perceive the old as in need of assessment and placement, as almost certainly suffering from organic brain syndrome, and therefore as untreatable. While some older persons do suffer from chronic organic brain syndrome, there are older schizophrenics, manic-depressives, and unipolar depressives as well as people with anxiety states, phobias, and adjustment disorders. All of these, if younger, would be seen as clearly suited to community mental health services. The old, however, tend to be tracked into case management, medication, and placement and away from acute inpatient treatment, day treatment, and outpatient therapies. In the change from one setting to another, with the consequent relabeling of problems, the psychotic elderly have most often been ignored and even assumed not to exist.

The preceding discussion has argued from history that certain of the elderly have been the responsibility of the mental health system or would be recognized as such if they were younger. Another approach begins with a different question but ends with a converging answer. In an attempt to become more clear about the nature of the elderly who are at risk of institutionalization, Lower-Walker and I (1985) reviewed the records of five hundred "at risk" elderly seen by a mobile geriatric mental health team. We categorized these frail elderly into seven groups: (1) those with medical disorders producing functional disability in the Activities of Daily Living (ADL) or Instrumental Activities of Daily Living (IADL) sense (e.g., persons with emphysema who are unable to walk well); (2) persons with Alzheimer's disease and other memory-impairing illnesses; (3) persons with other mental disorders (e.g., schizophrenia, paranoia, depression, and so on); (4) persons with behavior dangerous to others; (5) those with behavior dangerous to self (e.g., suicidal, severe self-neglect); (6) those with bizarre behavior, including annoying police, social workers, and so forth; and (7) persons whose social support system was inadequate to begin with or has broken down under stress (e.g., persons without family supports and those whose available support persons are themselves physically or mentally disabled). Clearly, this is a diverse group of subcategories of older people, and each category is likely to require a separate response to minimize the risk to inappropriate institutionalization. As listed, these problems would seem to call for intervention by medical treatment and rehabilitation, mental health treatment, community support, social control systems, and the dementia care system, if any exists.

It is worth noting in passing that even this listing of frail elderly fails to take into account the important fact that the cause of institutionalization often lies outside of the patient: caregiver illness or burden, family politics, financial problems, the lack of availability of needed support services, and the availability of institutional beds (Blumenthal 1980; Morycz 1980; Knight and Lower-Walker 1985; Nardone 1980).

Of these seven groups, not all are the responsibility of mental health treatment personnel. Persons with functional mental disorders would generally be accepted as primary responsibilities of the mental health system as would those who are dangerous to self and others and those with bizarre behavior if these behaviors are due to mental disorder. The memory-impaired elderly present a more complex problem in that mental health policy varies from state to state, with some including and others excluding the organic brain syndromes from the mental health domain of responsibility. (Similar discrepancies exist for the inclusion or exclusion of alcoholism and other substance abuse and developmental disabilities.) Recognizing this responsibility raises questions about the relationship of the mental health system to those other parts of the network of services for the elderly.

INSTITUTIONAL CARE AND THE ELDERLY

Deinstitutionalization in mental health has been coincident with the creation and proliferation of nursing homes (partly funded by Medicaid and intended to reduce long-term stay in acute medical hospitals) and residential care for the elderly (partly supported by Social Security/Supplemental Security income supports and intended as homes for frail elderly), all of which started in the 1960s. Programs were developed to redirect older patients from state hospitals to nursing homes, with or without a stay in the psychiatric ward of a local hospital (e.g., Rypins and Clark 1968; Ruffin and Urquhart 1980). Similarly, programs have been advocated to direct patients from nursing homes to residential care homes (Sherwood and Morris 1983;

Ruchlin and Morris 1983). In these studies, the residential care facility is seen as "community-based care" because it is non-medical, although many are at least as institutional in physical appearance and social organization as are nursing homes. In regard to the prevention of institutionalization of older clients, the question can be raised as to which level of institutional care is the target.

The notion of a range of care settings can organize our thinking about how institutional various institutions are. Knight and Lower-Walker (1985) proposed two conceptually and legally separate systems of care for the elderly. The long-term care system for the elderly as defined by licensing regulations moves from independent living to residential care, locked residential care, intermediate care, skilled nursing care, and locked skilled nursing care. The psychiatric system could be viewed as including acute psychiatric hospitals, state hospitals, and locked skilled nursing facilities. We noted several problems in considering either range to be a progressive hierarchy. First, patients enter and leave the system and move from level to level in a wide variety of ways. Our concept may be one of gradual deterioration and progressive movement up the scale, but reality fails to fit this image. For example, dementia patients who also have behavior problems may move from independent living to high levels of locked care and then move to more "independent" levels of care as their condition deteriorates and they are no longer capable of causing trouble. Second, for families, distance can play a major role in the perception of facilities as institutional; a state hospital close to home may be preferable to a nursing home placement further away. Third, the availability of treatment changes both the perception and possibly the legal status of institutional care. In the mental health system, it has been held that treatment is provided in exchange for loss of freedom (*O'Connor* v. *Donaldson* 1975; *Wyatt* v. *Stickney* 1971). In general, rehabilitation facilities, Alzheimer's special care units, and some actively treatment-oriented psychiatric facilities may seem less institutional than the average nursing home.

To further complicate the picture, home care is not necessarily equivalent to freedom and self-determination. The family may be better able to control and physically restrain than does any regulated facility. Home health and other community care agencies are relatively unregulated mainly because it is difficult to do surprise on-site inspection, and the care and degree of control may depend greatly on the individual worker.

The rationale for movement within the two systems is also different. Movement within the aging long-term care system is based on physical frailty and functional ability in the ADL sense. Movement within the psychiatric system is based on the degree of acuity of the psychiatric disorder and/or the overtness of behavioral problems. Problems arise when psychiatric staff fail to take physical problems or functional ability into account and when mental health workers, who tend to be more blasé about behavioral deviancy, are perceived by aging service providers as uncaring or arbitrary. The power of the mental health facility to lock doors and to enforce involuntary treatment may be envied by workers in the aging care system, and the decisions to accept some patients and reject others often appear arbitrary to those who are untrained in diagnosis or unfamiliar with the legal issues involved. Thus two interlocking but conceptually distinct systems with built-in tensions exist and are bound together by serving some of the same patients and many similar patients. Mental health patients, former mental health patients, and the cognitively impaired inhabit all of the levels of care in both systems. The presumed goal for the community mental health worker would be to seek the level of placement required by the patient's condition and to avoid unnecessarily restrictive placement.

COMMUNITY-BASED CARE AND THE OLDER AMERICANS' ACT

While not providing a different level of care, a different range of programs has developed over the same period of time, largely funded by or at least encouraged by the Older Americans' Act and the set of planning and coordination agencies funded by that act (the Administration on Aging, state Units on Aging, and Area Agencies on Aging). With a goal similar to that of the community mental health movement, this system and its funded services strive to keep older people independent and in the community. In general, this principle is related more to prevention of inappropriate skilled nursing care and has a less clear stance on residential care. Senior recreation centers, multipurpose centers, congregate and home-delivered meals, social model day care for adults, legal aide, in-home supportive services, volunteer support, and the long-term care ombudsman programs are all part of this system.

Until recently, neither mental health problems nor the needs of the demented were explicitly addressed by this system, and the recent changes in the authorizing legislation to mandate these interests have come at a time when funding has leveled out or is decreasing in the face of inflation. In spite of limited formal cooperation (Fleming et al. 1986), community mental health clients do get served in senior service sites, most often without being explicitly recognized as such.

Given the historical coincidence of the two approaches to prevention of institutionalization, it is of interest that there appears to be little concern that the aging system will duplicate the mistakes of the mental health system and contribute to the closing of institutional care while not providing adequate funding for the needed quantity and quality of community based care to cover the needs of those who are truly at risk.

The two systems espouse different approaches to prevention of institutionalization. The mental health system tends to favor community-based treatment, while the aging network argues for increased coordination of (presumably) existing services. The next section examines the mental health system's possible contributions to prevention of institutionalization of the elderly. For more explanation and critique of the aging network approach, works by Estes (1979) and Frankfather (1977) are recommended.

MENTAL HEALTH AND PREVENTION OF INSTITUTIONALIZATION OF THE AGED

In this mélange of problems and with this range of placements that are not always considered part of the mental health system of care, why would mental health approaches work in preventing unnecessary institutionalization of older people at risk? Taking the "at risk" groups defined above one at a time, let us consider possible answers to this question.

For the functionally impaired older person with medical problems, medical and rehabilitative treatments are likely to be primary, with mental health playing a supportive role. To the extent that depression and anxiety hinder recovery, interfere with compliance with treatment regimes, and produce increased disability, health psychology and behavioral medicine approaches will be important even with those persons for whom the medical cause of disability is certain. In many cases, the etiology of disability is likely to be uncertain or thought to be a mix of physical and psychological factors. In these cases, the role of the mental health team becomes even more important.

The older person with dementia is often claimed by neither medicine nor mental health but accounts for a large part of the long term care population. Increasingly, there are moves to create a separate system of care for the dementia patient. Much (although not all) of dementia care would seem to consist of a combination of behavioral intervention and psychotropic medication, which has historically been defined as mental health treatment.

Certainly, for the older person with mental disorders such as schizophrenia, paranoia, and depression, the role of the mental health system ought to be a fairly clear extension of work with younger adults with the same disorders. The propensity of mental health professionals to misdiagnose these disorders as senile dementia (see Settin 1982) or to rediagnose persons with lifelong histories of psychosis as being demented on the attainment of a certain age is simply an evasion of responsibility.

For elderly who are dangerous to themselves in the sense of being actively suicidal, the response should be similar to that for younger people. However, the reality is that the prejudice against the old is sufficiently prevalent that many feel that the desire of a 70-year-old to commit suicide is reasonable whereas that same desire at 32 is senseless and tragic. There may be more suicides for good reasons in late life, but common sense suggests that those who come to the attention of mental health professionals are uncertain about their desire and deserve professional attention. Other types of dangerousness to self in late life are more problematic. Many elderly are sufficiently ill to be able to commit suicide passively by withdrawing from medical care. The question of when this is evidence of depression and of when the patient is competent to make this decision and has the right to make it in certain circumstances is the center of an intense cyclone of legal, moral, and medical/psychiatric debate. In many social service systems, the demented older person can be described as dangerous to self because of serious self-neglect. This description is also a judgment call and one for which the legal rules vary considerably from place to place.

Behavior dangerous to others and bizarre behavior both tend to draw attention to the role of mental health professionals in social control. In these situations, the mental health professional often occupies an intermediary role between the police and courts, on the one hand, and families or formal social support systems, on the other. Again, the legal rules vary from place to place as do community standards of bizarre behavior. The best approach for the mental health professional is to find, if possible, treatable disorders and humane solutions while avoiding becoming a tool in others' power struggles and avoiding bypassing the due-process protections of the courts.

Social system breakdown brings into play the mental health system's ability (ideally) to intervene at levels other than those directly concerned with the identified patient. Often it is caregiver depression or other caregiver stress that makes the difference between community care and placement (Zarit, Orr, and Zarit 1985; Poulschock and Deimling 1984). In those instances, family therapy or therapy with the caregiver rather than the "patient" will be the effective strategy. When other breakdowns in support are implicated, the mental health professional may be able to shift into a consultant role and thereby enable the care system to function more adequately (Knight 1986a).

This brief overview highlights some of the potential roles for mental health professionals in preventing unnecessary institutionalization of older people by using theory- and practice-based interventions that are traditionally seen as part of mental health practice with younger adults. Historically, these methods have not been readily extended to older adults. This concern with the lack of availability of treatment-oriented approaches to the older client returns us to the concern of the first part of this chapter with barriers to treatment for the more acutely disordered older person. In this sense, both the short-term depressed older client and the long-term mentally ill client are likely to need a more aggressive outreach approach, although the services received after contact is made may very well differ. The next section discusses typical approaches to work with the elderly in community mental health.

TRADITIONAL OUTREACH TEAMS IN MENTAL HEALTH

When mental health services have been provided to older persons, the emphasis has been on assessment and making decisions about the older person (Zinberg 1964). Even though most such programs have adopted the Older Americans' Act rhetoric of prevention of institutionalization, the actual activities of the programs tend to operate within a framework of custodialism. Three common models of traditional service to the elderly include assessment and placement, assessment and referral, and the nursing home consultation team.

Assessment and Placement

In part as a result of the more general move of the mentally ill out of state psychiatric hospitals and into "the community," several locales have provided geriatric services that do assessment and placement. Depending on the composition and expertise of the team, the assessments can range from fairly rudimentary functional assessments that determine where in the range of residential environments the person can function to rather sophisticated mental status exams that attempt to define the patient's diagnosis more precisely. In either case, the team functions primarily as a gatekeeper in the local system of residential environments for the elderly and primarily screens people for admission to the psychiatric part of that system. Such programs have tended to define success in terms of where the patients end up living—in terms, for example, of numbers diverted from state hospital to nursing homes (Rypins and Clark 1968; Ruffin and Urquhart 1980). In fact, in these reports the diversion has been dramatic in numbers, decreasing geriatric commitments per year from 486 to 3 in a three-year time period. The principles were also laudable: to secure more appropriate treatment closer to home for the organic brain syndrome patient and to secure more acute treatment closer to home for the geropsychiatric patient.

Although usually viewed in more positive terms as leading to appropriate use of less restrictive levels of care, in some settings such teams can also be viewed as blocking access to care that patients and/or families may see as more desirable and that may, in fact, have higher staffing levels, more expertise, and be more treatment-oriented than are the more community-based settings. This becomes a problem particularly when applied at several levels of the system at once. In any event, the patients are usually viewed as passive elements in this system with no desires, decisions, or viewpoints of their own.

Assessment and Referral

Once the majority of former geriatric mental health patients were removed from the state hospital to nursing homes and residential care homes, the focus of the geriatric team shifted slightly from assessment and placement to assessment and referral. The concept for this model adheres closely to the information and referral model of the Older Americans' Act and can be seen as reflective of the Nixon era emphasis on getting government out of service provision and into a consultative and coordinative role (Estes 1979). The key assumption in such a model is that there are, in fact, a rich variety of other service providers to which clients with identified needs can be sent for assistance. This assumption is often violated and tends to be less and less true with the steady shrinking of governmental and private support for programs during the 1980s.

Without appropriate referrals, the team function can disintegrate into a focus on assessment for its own sake. While it can be helpful to receive an accurate assessment and information related to prognosis, services that would be useful, and so forth, it is also frustrating for staff, client, and family to confront the fact that needed and desired services are generally nonexistent, expensive, or scheduled in less than helpful ways. As the numbers of programs offering assessment and referral increase (including social services, mental health services, home health agencies, and a host of community-based aging programs), older persons and their families can be subjected to a bewildering variety of assessments that in many cases all lead to the same description of the paucity of locally available resources.

The potential problems of such an approach can be seen in the description by Wasson and Associates (1984) of an assessment and referral team. They comment on the strong relationship between client improvement and the willingness of the client or client's family to act on recommendations as well as on the problems in securing psychotherapy for all clients except those with access to home-delivered therapy provided by other agencies. While a good example of this type of team, these candid self-evaluations reveal the essential helplessness of the assessment and referral team.

Nursing Home Consultation Teams

One response to the move of large numbers of mentally ill elderly from psychiatric institutions to long-term care health facilities has been the provision of mental health consultation to nursing facilities. In the nursing home, both the psychotic and the demented elderly at times present behavior problems that are not easily tolerated or may pose a danger to staff and other residents. In areas without consultation teams, these problems will likely lead to admission to a psychiatric hospital or to transfer to another nursing home. A good consultation team can maintain the elderly patient in the original facility through staff consultation, behavior management, and use of psychotropic medication. A less than optimal team (such as described by Frankfather 1977) may consult strictly regarding medication, and when this fails, it may serve as a mobile admission unit to the psychiatric hospital or as the hospital's agent in refusing such admission.

While reflecting different approaches to providing mental health services to the elderly, these three models share some assumptions that are typical of traditional mental health programming for the elderly:

1. Most teams provide only assessment. Assessment is, of course, quite important with respect to the elderly, and mental health has a major potential role to play in differentiating dementia, delirium, depression, schizophrenia, paranoid states, anxiety states, and other common problems. But assessment should have a purpose and should be tightly linked to treatment or problem resolution.

2. The older client is generally assumed to be passive and not a part of the decision-making process. Staff or, in some cases, family guide the actual decision-making. In the worst cases, the decision is preordained by system-level economic decisions, and the assessment is mainly a smoke-screen—as when, for example, an expensive service like geropsychiatric hospitalization is going to be closed and so an assessment team is set up to guide people to other resources or to tell them that home care is preferable.

3. Related to the preceding point but conceptually different is the fact that older people are often assumed to be demented and therefore incompetent to participate in either decision-making or treatment. This assumption may be either explicit, as in the definition of all older people as having

organic brain syndrome, or implicit, as in the statement that they are "just old" where this description implies forgetfulness and incompetence. In hospital policy this assumption can be reflected in rediagnosing life long schizophrenics as demented when they reach a certain age and by considering 45-year-old patients with other neurological impairments as "geriatric cases."

4. The failure to attempt treatment and especially psychotherapeutic or psychosocial treatment of any kind reflects a therapeutic nihilism that is common in traditional programming for the elderly. Most systems of thought about mental health treatment argue that nothing can be done for the brain-impaired patient and that mental health professionals can hardly be expected to make the "just old" young again. Clearly, the development of any service program for older people depends on defining different working assumptions for at least some of our aged population.

The approach described in the remainder of this book takes from the existing team models the concern for accurate assessment and good referrals as well as the emphasis on the delivery of services to the client in the home environment whenever necessary. The critique of traditional services and the history of positive experiences in using psychotherapy as a change technique with older adults led to the decision to incorporate active psychotherapeutic services in the program model as the intervention strategy to achieve change as desired by the client. Psychotherapy was also seen as a possible strategy for minimizing inappropriate use of institutional care (defined here as either using twenty-four-hour care when living at home is still possible or using higher than needed levels of care). Finally, the existing teams also highlight the importance of providing good assessment and referral to older clients for the health and social services that they will also need because of their multiple coexisting problems. These assessment and referral services necessitate a good relationship with other components of the network of aging services.

SUMMARY

At the beginning of this chapter, questions were asked that can now be provisionally answered. How many of the elderly need mental health services? The answer is far from clear but is likely to be in the range of 7% to 20%, with most in this range having acute, treatable problems (e.g., depression, phobia). These figures should calm the fears of those who imagine existing resources being overwhelmed by huge numbers of older people with untreatable brain impairment. Do they underutilize mental health services in comparison with their need? Yes, but the difference may be less than we thought a decade ago, and improvements are already being seen. The problem of low use of services is also considered to be not unique to the elderly. Taken together, these observations suggest that the problem is not as large or as insurmountable as much of the literature suggests.

Why are services underutilized, and can we correct the underutilization? Briefly, the answers would appear to be in costs, physical inaccessibility, and therapists and potential clients who are largely uninformed about one another and about the benefits of psychotherapy for the elderly. Sliding-scale fees, greater public support (via Medicaid and Medicare) for outpatient and home-delivered mental health services, greater use of home visits, and enhanced education of therapists about assessment and therapy with the aged, combined with public education to acquaint the elderly with psychological problems and the benefits of mental health services as they now exist, are potential solutions.

Which elderly need services? Clearly not all of them. But there are older people who fit traditional concepts of mental health clients: older people who are depressed, anxious, phobic, paranoid, and schizophrenic and those who are dangerous to self or others or acting bizarrely due to mental disorder. There are others whose cases are perhaps less clear but who still could benefit from mental health intervention: the memory impaired elderly and more especially their families, who suffer greatly from the stress of caregiving, older people with physical illness or disability complicated by psychological factors, and those elderly with inadequate or overwhelmed support systems.

How can mental health services fit into the larger system of care for older adults? By outreach, consultation, and education, mental health services, which themselves span a wide range of institutional and community-based services, can offer something and can gain something at all levels of the complex range of aging services.

The next chapter takes us from the general and abstract to the application of these principles in the development of a mobile geriatric outreach team in a southern California county.

2

Beginning of Senior
Outreach Services

The preceding chapter considered the principles for an approach to provide outpatient mental health services to older people. What happens when these principles are applied to the development of a geriatric outreach team in a specific community? This chapter describes the application of these principles in developing an outreach program for the elderly in Ventura County, California.

Before describing the program itself, a few words about the locale in which it developed are appropriate. Ventura County is an urban southern California county, immediately north of Los Angeles County on the Pacific Coast, with a population of more than 600,000. During the years the program was developing, the county was experiencing rapid population growth, with the population of the elderly growing about twice as fast as the remainder of the population. The census of persons over 60 increased from approximately 60,000 in 1980 to an estimated 85,000 in 1985. (Estimated representation in the total population increased from 9% to 12% in that period.) The population increases come from both outmigration from the Los Angeles metropolitan area and from people moving to the county from other U.S. states. There are ten incorporated cities in the county, and they vary widely in size and in demography. The cities in the eastern county are contiguous with Los Angeles and identify more with L.A., whereas other cities have distinctive identities as small towns and even as rural communities. Ethnically, the county is predominately white, non-Hispanic. Hispanics comprise about 25% of the total population, with other sizable minorities of blacks, Asians, and Filipinos. About 9% of the elderly are Hispanic, while less than 2% of elderly are in the other minority groups.

Ventura was one of the first counties in California to participate in the state-funded mental health services system when it was created in 1956. Since that time, it has often been characterized by a willingness to try new models of care. In addition to the program for the elderly described in this book, Ventura County Mental Health had an extensive set of services for the chronically mentally ill in the mid-1970s and developed a comprehensive, integrated service system for mentally disordered children in the mid-1980s as part of a special state initiative.

The Ventura County approach to outreach to the elderly began in the late 1970s in response to the first signals that community mental health would switch from a more generic outreach to low-income persons in need of mental health services to a more targeted special-populations approach. At that time (1977) it was estimated that 2% of the outpatient client population was over 60 years of age. Rather than an immediate move to service provision, the Mental Health Department decided to prepare for such services with a twin strategy of inservice training for staff and community education for the senior population. These efforts recognized the mutual lack of understanding that then existed between mental health professionals and the elderly.

FORMATION OF A SENIOR OUTREACH PROGRAM

Inservice Training

The training effort, which lasted from 1978 to 1981, involved the planning and execution of four sessions per year that were oriented toward mental health staff but were open to interested people in other agencies as well. This openness to other senior service providers created a positive side effect of further reinforcing the role of the mental health center as an interested party in developing senior services locally as well as increasing interaction and referrals between mental health and other agency staff. The topics were varied and included basic information in gerontology was well as more specific mental health topics such as life-stage developmental models for therapy, the accurate diagnosis of dementia, and descriptions of existing models of mental health outreach to the elderly. The trainers for these sessions were from two sources: the Andrus Gerontology Center at the University of Southern California (about sixty miles away) had a grant to provide such training and was a source for academic gerontology expertise. More clinically oriented persons were recruited from the southern California region and represented clinicians who had some specialized work experience in aging or who "had an interest in gerontology."

While the training program was never formally evaluated, it appears that a number of positive objectives were realized. The training series clearly communicated the message that older people were becoming an important focus of departmental interest. Mental health staff at all levels and across the range of services provided were told by academic gerontologists that aging did not necessarily imply severe cognitive impairment or physical deterioration. Staff were also exposed to clinicians who had worked with a wide variety of kinds of older people and who had found this work successful, valuable, and interesting. Finally, staff in fact learned state-of-the-art aging and mental health techniques and information. The training sessions also provided opportunities for mental health staff who were working with older people to exchange information and views and to provide one another with support for what they were doing. This support was not always available from colleagues or program managers at each worker's home site.

From the viewpoint of a participant observer during the final stages of the training, there were some aspects that are worthy of note, illustrating as they do important points about the training process and the relationship between gerontology as an academic discipline and the clinical practice of gerontology. At that time (1979–1981), there were virtually no trainers available who had both academic training and clinical experience. The academic trainers were generally knowledgeable about the well elderly and focused mostly on "demythologizing" the aging process. While this perspective was valuable at first, there was a need in subsequent lectures to move to more sophisticated levels of theory and information and also to bridge the gap between descriptions of well elderly and the very real problems of the older people in mental health centers who are likely to be physically ill or disabled, depressed, chronically mentally ill, or demented.

Moreover, the clinicians available at the time generally had little or no formal education in gerontology and had knowledge based on their own experience, which was usually with one and only one of the following groups: outpatient clients with depression, chronically mentally ill in a large hospital setting (state hospital or Veterans' Administration), or demented elderly. In general, however, these presenters failed to appreciate the limits of their experience and generalized from these specific subgroups to the elderly in general and at times to the developmental process of aging. It was extremely rare to find people whose specialized interest or experience with older people constituted more than a small percentage of their professional practice. In many cases "older" outpatient cases were clients between 50 and 65. While the experience of these individuals was often interesting and even inspirational, it lacked a broader context of relationship to theory, knowledge, or other practitioners' experience.

Especially in the last year of the series, it became difficult to find people from either academia or the professional sector who could present information that would be new to this audience or who had more experience than some of the audience members who themselves had worked with small numbers of older people for a few years. It is unfortunate that many inservice trainers appeared to be convinced that they were addressing novices and that post-degree professionals with several years clinical experience were less intelligent and knowledgable than first-year graduate students.

Community Education and Outreach

Concurrently with the training effort for staff, the community education and outreach project was implemented. The cornerstone of this early effort was a series of educational workshops planned by the mental health center and entitled "Creative Aging Workshops" This title and the general emphasis of the workshops was on a positive and life-enhancing model of education for older adults rather than on a loss-deficit corrective model of service (see Reinhart and Sargent 1980, who describe these workshops in greater detail).

There were several important consequences of the planning process itself. Because the workshops were intended to cover a wide variety of topics, the planning process involved people from a number of different groups: several mental health department programs, public and private programs for older people, and active senior advocates. This experience of planning and carrying out a major community education effort naturally built interpersonal relationships among the involved providers, and these tended to translate into better agency relationships and better referral contacts. The contact between service providers and senior advocates served as an important and immediate reminder that not all older people were as problem-ridden as clients tend to be. The advocates also reminded planners of basic issues that are important to the seniors who were the intended audience: physical accessibility of sites, acceptability of sites, access to public transportation, potential stigma attached to some topics, and so on.

The topics were chosen to cover a wide range of concerns of interest to older people and included such areas as nutrition, exercise, and financial matters. The approach to issues related to mental health began with a focus on making friends, loneliness, adjusting to being a widow or widower, assertive training, and information contrasting normal aging and depression. A series of meetings were held over a period of four years and covered fifteen different sites throughout the county. All of the meetings were well attended and well received by participants. Most participants were the well elderly and aging service network providers. Many participants no doubt benefitted from the opportunity to discuss problems of their own or to learn more about mental health and other health topics. However, the longer lasting benefit of the programs was the image of the mental health department as an agency interested in seniors, the building of more personalized working relationships with other service providers, and the initiation of informal referrals. Thus, the well and active elderly could become comfortable and familiar with the department's services and departmental staff and with referring friends and relatives who have appropriate problems (or coming in themselves at later, more troubled times.)

Concurrently with the Creative Aging Workshops, the planning group, called the "Creative Aging Task Force," started meeting regularly. These meetings provided support for persons interested in working with older people and updates on developments in the system of services for older people and became a forum for planning and coordinating the department's future programming in the geriatric area. In the late 1970s, this group began advocating for the development of an outreach team that would provide an assessment and referral function. The team was planned to include a nurse, a social worker, and a rehabilitation therapist, and there was, consideration of adding a part-time psychologist to provide help with assessment and evaluation after the program had been running for a couple of years. At this point the department's intent was to copy the assessment and referral model described in chapter 1.

Senior Advocates and Program Development

The Creative Aging Workshops included senior advocates who from that time were integrally involved in providing advice and direction to the developing senior mental health program. The department had the good fortune to be in a community where senior advocates had taken an interest in mental health services to the extent that representation of elderly persons on the Mental Health Advisory Board was always substantial. Moreover, historically, leaders in the Mental Health Advisory Board often became leaders in the County Council on Aging and vice versa. Senior advocates were instrumental from early planning stages on in arguing for senior services being located at a site away from the central mental health offices where the inpatient and day treatment programs made clear the connection with mental illness. In addition, senior advocates reinforced the perceived need for home visits as a critical aspect of the services, and from experience, they were often able to point out drawbacks to plans that staff had not considered. For example, while nearness to bus lines was an obvious need, it was not clear to staff that some bus lines were themselves nearly inaccessible to seniors due to poorly planned connections and a limited number of exchange points among lines in the city.

The relationship was not, however, purely cooperative. In the early days in particular, senior advocates often took the position that mental health services were a frill and that the elderly needed more basic and "real" services. Or they would argue that older people neither needed or wanted mental health services, which would be stigmatizing to them anyway. In such instances, extensive effort was needed to educate, bargain with, or simply work around such opposition.

Training Phase 2: Intern Recruitment

In the late 1970s, the training officer had initiated a process of recruiting clinical psychology interns whose interests and academic preparation coincided with the outreach and program development goals of the Department. In 1978, an intern who had academic preparation in the aging field and was interested in clinical experience and training with the elderly was recruited. Training rotations included crisis programs, day treatment, and outpatient clinics. For each of these, a special effort was made to track older clients to the intern's caseload, and the personal contact with crisis team staff led to referral to outpatient services of some elderly who otherwise would not have been considered appropriate. The internship included a community services rotation (i.e., consultation and education), which in this instance involved an ongoing consultation with the city housing authority covering a wide range of psychosocial problems among the elderly as well as involvement with the Creative Aging Workshops and the Creative Aging Task Force. At the close of the predoctoral internship year, the impact of the intern on the department was largely limited to some increased awareness of the need for accurate diagnosis of the elderly and of the efficacy of psychotherapy with the elderly. The primary impact on planning was that the intern had shown that the widely accepted belief that no elderly person would consent to and complete paperwork and pay for outpatient therapy at standard sliding-scale fee rates was incorrect.

At the close of the internship year, a second-year postdoctoral internship training agreement was negotiated, with the same intern concentrating more effort in outreach to and clinical services for the aged. Outpatient caseload increased from about a 20% focus on elderly to an 80% focus, with intradepartmental consultations on assessment issues and staff training becoming a larger component of the postdoctoral training. In addition, there were specific projects, including the development of a videotape training film for potential elderly clients to explain the work of therapy and a research project on the influence of therapists' attitudes toward the elderly on their actual work with older clients. Increased visibility within and outside of the department led to a greater acceptance of the department's role in working with older people and provided a continuing platform for the advocacy of the importance of outpatient therapy in mental health plans for services to older clients. Toward the end of the postdoctoral year, it was also possible to demonstrate that the part-time clinical work of this one intern had doubled the proportion of elderly people seen in the department's outpatient clinics. This increase, while obviously a function of the paucity of elderly seen before the intern's arrival, still provided hard evidence that the goal of increased service to this group was one attainable with reasonable resources.

Toward the end of this postdoctoral year, after considerable advocacy and negotiation, the department changed its plans and used a grant of augmentation monies from the state Department of Mental Health to start up a senior outreach team that would include outpatient therapy, with field visits as a principal service component, along with assessment and referral and consultation and education. The team structure was changed to include the geropsychologist as coordinator, a mental health nurse, and a clinical social worker; A consulting psychiatrist was added soon after. Clerical support to help with the paperwork and collections that are part of outpatient clinic services was also added.

ISSUES IN THE FORMATION OF A SENIOR OUTREACH TEAM

The Decision to Offer Outpatient Therapy

As has been commented on several times above, the concept of providing outpatient therapy to older people was an idea whose time had not yet come in California in 1980. Existing outreach teams, the state department of mental health, keynote speakers at NIMH/Administration on Aging (AOA) sponsored conferences on mental health and aging, and aging advocates all argued that the elderly would not accept traditional mental health outpatient services. The historical basis and the rationale for the department's decision to opt for therapeutic optimism and extend mental health services to older people have already been described. It is worth noting that the decision also has important fiscal implications in that treatment services such as mental health assessment, psychotherapy, and psychotropic medication are generally seen by third-party payers as billable and therefore revenue-generating services. On the other hand, more traditional outreach teams, which rely on assessment and referral perhaps supplemented by case management often delivered by paraprofessionals, are virtually automatically a non-billable, non-income generating service whose total cost must be borne by the sponsoring agency. The decision to offer therapy and to do so in a clinically and fiscally sound manner also dictates the use of staff trained at the psychotherapeutic level and provided with clinical supervision by the clinical psychologist and psychiatrist on the team.

The Interdisciplinary Team

The Senior Outreach Team has always had representatives from psychology, psychiatry, clinical social work, and nursing on the clinical staff. The interdisciplinary nature of the service has required both some understanding of the unique contributions of each discipline as well as the development of a commonality of skills as applied gerontologists. To date, the roles have been much as follows:

Psychologist (in this case, clinical geropsychologist): Team manager, clinically responsible for services delivered. Direct provision of assessment, psychological testing, psychotherapy, consultation, and education. Group supervision of team in once-a-week meeting. Individual supervision of mental health nurses and of as yet unlicensed staff and students. As geropsychologist, responsible for developing new staff's appreciation of differences and similarities in working with older people and for continuing education of staff about new information in the field.

Psychiatrist: Responsible for medication evaluations and medication management for clients' psychotropic medication. Liaison with medical profession. Initial medical and neurological screening of patients who have not seen physician in some time. Supervision of nursing assessments and of medical students and psychiatric residents.

Clinical Social Worker: Often the major providers of direct psychotherapy to clients. Responsible for day-to-day liaison with other agencies and for understanding of importance of life-span psychosocial histories.

Mental Health Nurses: Responsible for thorough assessments of clients, including mental status, nursing assessment of physical status, and medications. With supervision, provide ongoing therapy visits.

It cannot be overemphasized that the complex and interacting nature of older people's problems, which generally span medical, mental health, and social casework issues, requires not only the presence of members of different disciplines but also a collaborative, interactive style of work. In this model, all members of the team do home visits, and all members participate in initial and ongoing assessments. As team members do assessments in pairs and learn to work together, there is sharing of knowledge and skills and some blurring of disciplinary lines to the extent permissible by law and good sense. In this sense, nonmedical members of the team learn to recognize common warning signs or complaints that may represent true medical problems and become aware of medication side effects. All team members become skilled at memory assessment and at recognition of common psychological disorders in the elderly as well as developing an appreciation of one another's unique skills (e.g., some staff have proved especially perceptive at recognizing alcoholism or early signs of dementia without much clearly specifiable objective data but with follow-ups that prove them correct).

Given the apparent scarcity of programs in which persons of different disciplinary background collaborate and do, in fact, work as a team, a few words about the relative success of this approach are in order. From the earliest days of the program's development, it was clear to me that we must blend together our different backgrounds and actively function as a team in order to help the elderly with their complex needs and to prevent the members of the program from being overwhelmed by those parts of their clients' problems that they were personally unprepared to handle. In looking backward, I can identify certain principles that were helpful in developing team spirit.

In general, negative stereotyping of other disciplines has been actively discouraged, and persons voicing such feelings have been encouraged to consider counterbalancing strengths of other team members. Most of us form part of our professional identity by being taught negative qualities of other disciplines. This negative stereotyping works up the hierarchy as well as down. Regardless of the truth of particular statements, they contribute nothing to team spirit or to the solution of clients' problems.

Along these same lines, team members have always been encouraged to keep the client's interest in the foreground. Problems are bound to arise, but the principle for solving them should be: What's good for the client?

When problems have arisen, their resolution has been a high priority for myself as team manager. This means that individuals are encouraged to work problems out with one another, and if that proves impossible, to meet with me until a disagreement is resolved. Intrastaff conflicts can only worsen if ignored.

When possible, staff have been selected with consideration given to their likely impact on team functioning. Working with a multiple-problem population is difficult enough without adding personal conflict among staff to the difficulty.

The staff met weekly to discuss clients and team functioning, and most staff met individually with the program manager on a weekly basis to discuss clients and program issues. There were frequent ad hoc meetings among involved staff to discuss client problems as needed. These meetings not only dealt with case management issues and conflict resolution but also often involved mutual clinical supervision. This mutual supervision is important to deal with countertransference issues and the emotional hazards of work with older adults, such as grieving for clients who die. (Chapter 7 discusses emotional hazards in more detail.) This level of communication is essential to a geriatric outreach team. A "private practice" model (which is also typical of many public clinics) of individual responsibility for clients is not workable with this population.

The Mix of Services

The early model of team organization and services recognized the need for assessment to clarify the nature of the presenting problem, treatment of treatable mental health problems, and outreach and education to assist in casefinding and also to improve the overall sophistication of services to the elderly as related to mental health and aging.

Assessment: The assessment process has always relied heavily on open-ended clinical interviewing that allows for individual tailoring of the assessment to the presented problem and the apparent needs of the potential client. This assessment follows an outline, however, and includes some review of medical history and medications, a mental status assessment including both cognitive and emotional status, a review of the family system and of current and past attempts to utilize the local network of services to seniors, and a reanalysis of the presented problem. An accurate assessment is the sine qua non of geriatric service delivery. Inaccuracy in the assessment process is quite likely to lead to the intervention doing more harm than good. This assessment process concludes with a referral, a crisis intervention, or an explanation of the nature of outpatient services and their application to this specific problem.

Therapy: The therapeutic process has included both psychotherapy and psychotropic medication as judged to be necessary by the client and the outreach team. While therapy is open-ended and in some instances has lasted for years, the mean for all cases has been about eight to twelve sessions. Most therapy visits (about 55%) have taken place in the client's home. After the first three to four months, most clients are seen every two weeks. Some clients are started on this biweekly schedule.

Mental Health and Aging Education: Viewed in part as a continuation of the department's twofold educational approach to teach potential clients about mental health services and to train mental health staff and other providers in the aging services system to a higher level of sophistication about the mental health needs of the elderly and in part as an outreach and casefinding method, education has been an important outreach team function. In the early years, more than 50% of the team's time was spent in mental health education, consultation, and promotion efforts, but in recent years, as the program has become well known and solidly established in the community, these activities have dwindled to 20%.

Funding

A major consideration in initiating any program is funding. Ventura County Mental Health was able to use a variety of funding sources in starting and maintaining the program described here, and much of the creative work that could be done was enabled by the unusual stability of these sources. California has a program of state-funded public mental health services under the Short-Doyle Act. The original start-up money for Senior Outreach and the assurance of continuing funding came from augmented funding to the basic budget that had to be spent on a priority population group. California also supplements federal Medicaid to a generous level in the mental health benefit package, and Medi-Cal payments for eligible clients have been an important source of funding. Medicare payments for the program as a hospital-based clinic (the Mental Health Department is closely affiliated with the county medical center) have been generous. Patient fees and private insurance have supplemented public funds but cover less than 5% of costs. (It is, however, my impression that the state mandated sliding scale is quite generous at some levels and that many of our clients could pay more and in fact some have asked to.) Over the years, outside sources of funding have covered 75% to 100% of program costs.

Research and Evaluation

The Ventura Team has included a research and evaluation component that has helped to guide our approach to outreach, to adapt our outreach strategies to changing program needs, and to change service strategy as needed. There is so little known about mental health and aging at this point that the ability to analyze our own efforts has been highly important in our development. This research program (described in the second section of this book, chapters 8–11) has helped us to learn continually from our own experience and to change program direction as needed.

SUMMARY

The description given in this chapter has taken the principles developed in chapter 1 and shown how they were exemplified in the development of the Ventura County Senior Outreach Team. The next several chapters explore further the component services of outreach to the elderly in community mental health, continuing to draw on the experiences of the Ventura County Team. One question that will be on the mind of many readers is to what extent the Ventura County experience can be generalized to other localities.

Are the elderly different here? The question is impossible to answer specifically. Later research chapters contain more specific information on our clients. It is not my impression that the Ventura County elderly seen by a county mental health department were on the whole very much more educated or sophisticated about mental health than people I have met in other parts of the country (having been raised and educated in Arkansas and Indiana). Many of our clients have been relatively uneducated, and some have been non-English speaking immigrants from Mexico (see chapter 11).

Judging from discussions with geriatric mental health workers in other states and other California counties, one tremedous benefit that we had was the active involvement of some senior advocates in the mental health advisory board. This was true for years before I became involved there, and I have no idea why this happens in some areas and not in others, aside from the non-helpful speculation that it depends on individual interests of individual advocates.

The other principle difference was the administrative support for the concept, which was there from the beginning. As noted at the beginning of the chapter, Ventura County has a history of innovation in mental health services. This background and the specific interests of individual administrators made a great deal of difference in starting the program and one that I have discovered largely in retrospect as I have encountered other managers in other locales who are as committed to blocking the development of programs for the elderly as those in Ventura County are to promoting them. As will be seen in chapter 8, research also supports the importance of management variables and commitment of resources to this work in order to overcome the presumed "barriers to services" for the elderly.

As stated earlier, a good assessment is the backbone of all intervention with the elderly. The next chapter describes the development of an assessment program in community mental health.

3

Developing the
Home Visit Assessment

The key element of any outreach team model is the assessment visit. While early visits in fact serve purposes other than assessment, such as establishing rapport with the client and providing a context for educating the client about the value of psychotherapy, the focus of this chapter is the nature of the assessment itself. The elderly are widely recognized to be a population with multiple problems and one in which a wide variety of problems generally coexist within the same person. These problems are likely to include medical, mental health, and social casework needs. I have argued elsewhere (1986a, 1983) that mental health services lie conceptually between medical and social services and that one purpose of a mental health assessment is to clarify what services within this continuum each individual client actually needs. The complexity of both the problems of older people and their service network combine to make it less likely that older people will themselves correctly select appropriate services and service providers.

There are also complex issues of diagnosis within the range of potential mental health disorders that older people may present. The greater prevalence of illnesses among the elderly make it more likely that emotional distress can be the result of physical rather than psychological processes. The number of medications taken by the elderly raises the probability of emotional distress due to medication effects. Conversely, the tendency of diseases to be present with nonspecific nonacute symptoms and the tendency of the elderly to describe emotional distress in more somatic language make it likely that psychological distress may be mistaken for physical illness. Both clinical and training experiences suggest that with the elderly physicians tend to ascribe problems to psychological causes, while psychologists ascribe them to physical causes.

As is usually true of physical disorders in the elderly, the lines between different mental disorders appears less clear than among younger adults. The increased prevalence of diffuse organic mental disorders in older people further complicates the diagnostic process by making some degree of competence in cognitive assessment and neuropsychology a virtual necessity. The higher likelihood of irreversible cognitive impairment in late life (primarily Alzheimer's disease and multi-infarct dementia) poses the necessity of screening for neurological problems that are quite difficult to diagnose and of determining whether the cognitive impairment means that therapy will need modification or simply be impossible. Differential diagnosis among dementia, delirium, depression, anxiety, and psychosis are notoriously difficult among older people (Knight 1986a; Zarit 1980).

Furthermore, the picture is complicated by the need to assess functional competency in older people. Most decisions regarding appropriate living arrangements and need for in-home supportive services depend more on functional ability than on the presence or even the severity (from the clinical standpoint) of disorders. Given the same disorders, two older people may function at quite different levels. In many cases, an assessment of abilities to eat, use the toilet, bathe, walk, pay bills, buy groceries, and so forth becomes more important than clinical diagnosis.

Even given similar levels of functional ability, true disability may depend on a variety of environmental elements, including presence of family, the health of family interactions, the richness of the community's supportive service system, the economic wealth of the individual, the health of the principal caregiver and so on (Blumenthal 1980). In this sense, the question of person-environment fit becomes a major issue in the assessment.

Given this broad array of issues, the assessment needs to be interdisciplinary in nature; in fact, most assessment teams tend to include at least one person from a medical or nursing background and one from a psychosocial orientation. The actual functioning of the assessment team will also depend heavily on the organization for which the team works and the actual range of decisions that can be made given the resources of the community in which it works. The range of competencies needed are those typically associated with fields such as medicine, nursing, psychology, social work, and the rehabilitation therapies. Unless the team is located in a medical school or large regional medical center, it is unlikely that such expertise will be immediately available. In most community-based programs, the available disciplines will have to make do and may have to stretch into related areas of competency. Unless team members have specific expertise in aging, additional training is likely to be necessary, especially for the recognition of diffuse cognitive impairment in the elderly.

The complexity of the problems of frail older people requires that as much information as possible be obtained. Conducting the assessment in the home, which is likely to be necessary because of the client's condition and functional ability, also helps increase the available information. Involving other people such as the client's family and any other professionals from health care or social services, is also helpful and reduces the likelihood of mistakes and of various helpers working at cross purposes.

ROLE OF THE MENTAL HEALTH ASSESSMENT TEAM

Given the complexity of the services available in many communities, it is important to have a clear concept of what other assessments are available in the community and how these compare to what one's own program is proposing to do. This will help to prevent duplication of services, to define one's own program, and to avoid unduly annoying clients who are already ill and overburdened. In many communities, a relatively wide variety of assessments is available, including diagnostic evaluations by physicians and various home health agency assessments, which (especially after discharge from a hospital) are likely to include separate evaluations by a nurse, a social worker, and two or more rehabilitation therapists. In addition, a growing number of social work and aging services agencies are doing various types of assessments designed to connect elders in need to appropriate services.

Many agency assessments serve mainly to answer the question of whether the client is appropriate for that agency's services. All too often, when the answer is no, the agency has no well thought-out referrals to offer. The client may receive nothing, or perhaps worse, a few phone numbers of agencies that the referring agency knows have nothing to offer. It would seem more humane to offer an assessment only when there is a purpose for the assessment and at least a strong possibility that help will follow. For the mental health team, this issue forces consideration of the purpose and consequences of assessment: What, other than the assessment itself, does the team offer? For what purposes will the assessment be used if the team judges mental health treatment to be inappropriate?

For those who are not in need of mental health care, the assessment team must be able to relate observed deficits and social problems to appropriate available services in the community. In many instances, this will be a relatively straightforward task, simply involving referral of those who need meals to meal sites, those who need socialization to recreation centers, and so forth. A more creative problem-solving approach is called for when the client's needs do not match local resources. If a client needs transportation to a doctor out of the local area, for example, the team will need to explore resources in the family and perhaps make calls to arrange for an exception for this "special case" of need. This process takes the assessment team an extra step into active assistance of clients, connecting them to services for other than mental health needs.

Open-Ended Assessments

Faced with such complexity, the natural response of an assessment team is to attempt to organize the task into questionnaires, outlines, and the like and to impose fairly simple decision rules onto this organized information. Such attempts tend to organize the interview in a way that allows for very little personalized interaction with the client and very little adaptation of the format to his or her specific needs. Such information-gathering techniques are also often quite long, requiring several hours to complete adequately. Furthermore, fairly large components of questionnaires are often not related to the questions that need to be answered for that specific client or else the answers are fairly obvious without detailed questioning. (For example, some clients are obviously cognitively intact, and others are obviously severely cognitively impaired. In either case, a detailed mental status examination serves no real purpose for the client.)

An open-ended assessment interview has the advantages of starting with the client's definition of the problem, allowing for a pacing of the interview that is consistent with the client's abilities and needs, and permitting the interviewer to skip over areas that are of little concern and to explore in depth those areas that do pose problems for the client. The client is more likely to feel understood and less likely to feel evaluated or like a guinea pig. This "client friendly" approach is especially important in primary care and outreach-oriented settings, while being of less concern in long-term care institutions and tertiary care settings, where clients have more time and are committed to or available for lengthier diagnostic processes. In fact, especially in the first years of operation of the Ventura Team, staff discussed extensively the use of various assessment procedures, including psychological testing, in terms of the relative merits of the information to be gained from the assessment versus the likelihood of the procedure becoming a barrier to therapy for the individual clients. In the outreach setting, the client's view of any procedure must be considered and weighed against the true value of any information to be gained.

On the other hand, the open-ended interview is only as good as the interviewer conducting it. While most quality training programs produce an acceptable standard of ability in conducting assessment interviews within that profession, the need for multidisciplinary assessment in the elderly tends to produce errors in interviewers that are somewhat consistent. The following examples are admittedly stereotypical, but they do serve to illustrate this point. Medically oriented persons will tend to focus on medical symptoms and may miss emotional or social problems altogether or be relatively unable to distinguish among types of psychological disorders. Psychosocially oriented people, in contrast, may focus so much on mental aspects that they conclude that someone is fine, while that individual is in fact functionally disabled for physical reasons. Nurses and social workers tend to be more tuned into environmental cues and functional ability. Physicians and psychologists, on the other hand, tend to focus on relatively minute questions and diagnoses that depend less on observation and more on microlevel analysis. Thus, the physician will probe for why the patient cannot walk, the psychologist for differences between phobia and generalized anxiety.

Another aspect of interviewer bias lies in the level of care at which the interviewer was trained or has had most of his or her work experience. People who were trained in community-based programs tend to see a broader mix of clients in a range from normal to moderate and perhaps higher levels of severity in mental functioning. Persons trained in institutional settings tend to have experience with moderate to catastrophically impaired patients. Persons trained in tertiary care settings, such as university medical centers, tend to see diagnostically complex cases that have been screened at the primary and secondary levels and selected for training value. Each level creates its own skills and blind spots. For example, the community-based worker is most likely to be interested in level of cognitive impairment and functional ability as related to decisions to be made about use of different support programs and the need for institutional care. There is likely to be less interest in the cause of the impairment among, say, Alzheimer's disease, multi-infarct dementia, or Pick's disease. It is quite possible that the occasional older person with a rare but more treatable neurological disorder will not be picked up as he or she would be in a tertiary care setting. A worker trained in institutional care may become so adapted to working with high levels of disability that such a worker might see earlier levels as equivalent to normalcy, a stance that community-based workers and family members are not likely to agree with. A person trained in tertiary care settings may feel totally lost without using extensive (and expensive) tests and hours-long interviews in order to make decisions. These differences become problems, of course, principally when a person trained in one setting attempts to work in another one or to train people who work in a different setting.

As I have mentioned already, the open-ended assessment process for a mental health team needs to answer two classes of questions. Is the client in the right place? This question explores for medical problems, mental health concerns, and social service needs and aims for sufficient specificity to make an accurate referral or to give genuinely helpful advice to the client. If mental health needs are identified, the second class of question is what type of mental health problem does the client have? The answer needs to be specific with respect to diagnosis and degree of impairment, and it must help in planning the intervention and guiding its course until the next reevaluation. In many cases, there will be multiple mental health problems as well as medical problems and social needs, and the intervention plans will be appropriately complex.

The open-ended interview requires some ability to do initial screening in areas beyond the interviewer's principal areas of competence. For example, some questions about medical history and the last time the client was seen by a physician as well as observations of swelling of legs and ankles and ability to walk, see, and hear are essential. The most problematic area is the client's report of fatigue or general sense of dysphoria; these complaints can be related to a number of physical and a number of psychological disorders.

Similarly, everyone needs at least some guidelines as to when forgetfulness needs further evaluation. In both community- and institution-based programs, there is often tremendous reluctance to perceive forgetfulness as a problem or an explanation of other problem behavior. In addition to simple mental status questions there are behavioral patterns that probably indicate a need for more assessment. People who come to the office for an appointment on the wrong day or the wrong time of day, people who invite others into their home without any clear idea of who they are, people who return to an information and referral service for the same information without awareness of repetition, and people who answer questions vaguely. ("I don't pay much attention to time now"; "I haven't looked at the paper so I don't know today's date"; "I expect there's a war on somewhere"; "Well, I handle that problem just like anyone else would") are often giving an early signal. Reports from family members of failing ability are more often accurate than not and generally call for more evaluation.

There is also the need to evaluate medications in terms of what is taken rather than what is prescribed and also to evaluate nutrition in terms of what is actually eaten and/or in terms of observed loss in weight. Moreover, information should be obtained from other sources such as physicians, family, friends, and neighbors, where these are available and confidentiality allows access. Observation becomes important in noting level of grooming, neatness of the home (as compared to prior level as well as in terms of absolute judgments; one also one needs to be sure that the client, rather than family members, community agencies, etc., is currently doing the housekeeping), energy level, food on hand in the house, the presence of more medication bottles than medications being reported, presence of alcoholic beverages and so on. Such observations can go in either direction. I once had the opportunity to see the home of a long-term office visit client who had reported maintaining a very sloppy house as part of her depression only to observe that the house was in fact far neater than average.

The essential structure of open-ended interviews tends to be a decision-oriented, problem-solving conversation that "branches" into more detail in areas where client responses suggest more information is needed and skips lightly over areas where client responses or therapist observation suggest there is little to be gained from futher questioning. It is this adaptability that is both the strength and the weakness of the open-ended interview style. Obviously, such an assessment relies on interviewer skill and judgment, and this reliance may need to be modified by the addition of more structure.

In fact, this was the case in the Ventura Outreach Team, which did move to a more structured assessment. During the early part of the third year of operation, the team's functioning was evaluated by a medical sociologist who visited the team under the Gerontological Society's Summer Research Fellowship program. Her observations called attention to the discrepancies in information collected during initial assessment interviews even within our relatively close-knit multidisciplinary team. Each team member was more likely to ask and even more likely to write down some kinds of information to the exclusion of other types. For example, the psychologist was more likely to make a note of the client's mental status exam score and less likely than the nurses to write down that the client had amputated toes due to diabetes, even though both had and used all of the information in the first evaluation. Problems arose when the client would be reevaluated months later, and only individual recall was available to assess change.

This observation and the consultant's discussions with team members about this finding led to the introduction into the note-taking procedure of an outline structure that was not part of the formal record keeping system. Compliance with these changes was in large part motivated by the team's growing awareness that many contacts we had previously considered as one-time-only visits that did not need much systematic recording would, over periods of years, in fact become repeat contacts so that information from earlier visits would become very helpful.

The outline adopted consisted of the following headings: medical history, mental status, medications, family supports, social system supports utilized, living arrangement, outcome of visit. In addition, about a year later, staff made an effort to include conclusions about the existence and level of dementing illness as well as the results of structured mental status examinations if given. This outline provides a more standardized report of the interview while preserving the advantages of the open-ended assessment. It also provides the essential elements for deciding which medical, mental health, and social service needs the client has in order to develop an appropriate intervention.

STRUCTURED MENTAL STATUS EXAMS

The use of structured mental status exams for cognitive impairment deserves some discussion. There are a variety of such tests available. The most commonly used in community mental health centers appear to be the Kahn Mental Status Questionnaire (KMSQ), a ten-item exam, and the Folstein Mini-Mental Status Exam (MMS), a thirty-point questionnaire. Both rely mostly on verbal performance tasks and principally measure general fund of information. Both have some claim to demonstrated validity in measuring diffuse cognitive impairment of the sort caused by dementia of the Alzheimer's type. Both are best at picking up dementias of moderate or greater severity.

But early decline and even middle stages in bright, well-educated subjects is very difficult to assess with any available test. (In one instance, the team social worker referred a woman with a Ph.D. in English literature who had scored very well on the Folstein but still "seemed impaired" for more assessment. She did well on other tests of memory as well, even though she did not recall the social worker's name after five one-hour sessions, nor did she know what state she had lived in prior to moving in California. She was also unable to give any clear idea as to what the articles she had published in midlife were about.) Available mental status exams are also sufficiently limited in the scope of functions assessed such that localized impairment in the brain may be missed altogether, especially if the impairment involves primarily visuospatial processing or the use of visual cues to reach conclusions. We once had a client who consistently scored no errors on the KMSQ even though he could not tell whether it was day or night while looking out the window.

Neither test is well equipped to distinguish between cognitive decline due to brain impairment and cognitive impairment due to depression, schizophrenia, or other psychological disorder. Folstein himself points out that in this regard the best evidence is a treatment trial with repeated testing to determine whether the cognitive impairment changes with treatment of the depression (Folstein, Folstein, and McHugh 1975).

With these cautions in mind, these tests can provide an important index of progressive loss of functioning in those individuals for whom the test works. Evidence of decline and some sense of the rate of decline can be helpful to both the clinician and the family in planning for the client over a period of several years. It is also essential to look at other evidence, including functional ability, consistent recall of recent events and life history, and medical findings, and to push for a neurological consultation if verbal and nonverbal evidence is inconsistent (e.g., if the client does very well on general information and then cannot perform on the Face Hand Test or a figure drawing test).

DEVELOPMENT OF THE SENIOR OUTREACH MENTAL STATUS ASSESSMENT

The tests discussed above were judged to be restricted in scope of abilities tested, and the scores often added very little to what was apparent from clinical interview and the client's behavior. In addition, a primary concern of the Ventura Team clinical staff became the reduction of false negatives— that is, clients with scores in the normal range who turn out over time to have been in the early stages of dementing illness. There are two costs related to this type of error. The clinician often discovers after several months of psychotherapy that attempted to treat the emotional causes of social withdrawal, irritation within family, and so forth that the patient is, in fact, dementing. More importantly, family members experience considerable frustration and an increase in their distress when they are told that the client is not as impaired as they thought and can recover, only to have this sense of hope taken away again.

After attempts to use various other mental status exams and depression inventories, the Ventura Team developed the Senior Outreach Mental Status Assessment, that follows these guidelines: (1) several sense modalities should be involved to maximize the likelihood of catching deficits that affect one area of the brain more than another; (2) actual tests of memory in the cognitive processing sense should be utilized, with examples to tap immediate and delayed recall and also recognition memory included (see Kintsch 1970; Klatsky 1975; Craik and Trehub 1982); (3) competing hypotheses should be represented in the test battery, so that, say, a test of depression needs to be made and some measure of subjective complaints of memory needs to be ascertained. Although Zarit's (1980) assertion that memory complaints are related more to depression than to memory loss has been replicated in some studies but not in others (see, for example, Scogin, Storandt, and Lott 1985; Niederehe 1986; O'Hara et al. 1986.), there appears to be ample reason to consider and to measure performance, complaints and depression separately and to track them over time.

The assessment scale draws on two research reports and four previously published tests as item pools. The reports are the well-documented development of the Short-CARE protocol by Barry Gurland et al. at Columbia University (1984) and work on the use of recall and recognition tasks to differentiate early and late stages of dementia by Vitaliano et al. (1984) at the University of Washington Medical School in Seattle. The latter research drew on the Folstein Mini-Mental, the Wechsler Memory Scale, and the Mattis Dementia Scale. The Short-CARE was judged to be much too long for our purposes and so only the memory, subjective memory, and a reduced version of the depression scale are used. The Face Hand Test was also incorporated because of its reliance on somatosensory modality. The Short-CARE scales and the Face Hand Test are supplemented by a structured interview that uses the Digits Forward and Digits Backward Tests from the Wechsler Memory Scale (as tests of concentration) and the Logical Memory Test as test of delayed recall for prose. The questions from the Folstein Mini-Mental State that call for sentence construction, sentence repetition, recall of three objects, and following instructions are used. The "crossing out *A*'s" test and the tests of word and design recognition from the Mattis Dementia Rating Scale complete the interview.

Data is still being collected to check the psychometric properties of the Senior Outreach Mental Status Assessment (SOMSA) interview. Clinical impressions to date suggest that delayed recall items show considerable impairment long before memory items from the Short-CARE are missed and that this is usually congruent with family reports of reduced functioning at home as well as a worsening in cognitive functioning over time. For example, whereas several individuals with cases of possible depression reported by family members have presented no complaint of depressed mood or fatigue but have demonstrated withdrawal and reduced activity, mental status testing yielded only a failure in delayed recall. Follow-up over a period of years verified that the problem was progressive cognitive impairment rather than depression.

HOME VISIT ISSUES IN ASSESSMENT

As has been discussed before, the use of home visits is an essential part of the senior outreach team and is necessary to overcome barriers to physical and psychosocial accessibility. Few mental health providers are trained to provide home visits and often feel quite apprehensive about the impact of changing the setting from office to home on the quality of services rendered. Since the mental health assessment process is essentially verbal and does not require any heavy and non-transportable technical equipment, in principle anything that can be done in the office can be done at home. However, there are, of course, some modifications that are implied by the change of locale from the professional office to the client's home.

One of the most salient changes is that more and different information is available. In the office context, the client is the sole source of information about his or her functioning, ability to care for himself or herself and the home, relationships with others and so forth. This self-report can be distorted in either direction. Demented older people often blithely claim higher levels of functioning than is valid. Depressed clients may exaggerate deficiencies. For example, one client asserted there was no food in the house. When the kitchen was inspected (with permission), there was easily a week's supply.

In the home, there is opportunity to observe the client's life setting and often some opportunity to interview family, friends, and neighbors as they drop in or telephone. While the presence of the interviewer will make these visits different from the usual interaction, valuable information can be gained from observing these contacts. A home visit may reveal that "isolated" elderly have several impromptu visits from family and neighbors, that meal companions are actually delusions based on magazine covers, that a feared spouse is physically frail and barely able to walk, or that paranoid-sounding claims about being constantly watched by neighbors are an actual fact of life in a mobile home park or senior apartment complex.

The fact that the interview takes place in the client's home where others may be present or may drop in does mean that the context and content of the interview is less controlled and is subject to interruption. If the client is comfortable with others being included in the session and if the therapist is not overly rigid and can change styles to take advantage of chances for impromptu family sessions or to have sessions that may be part individual and part family therapy, then both the assessment and the treatment can move more smoothly and more quickly than in the more structured and controlled office environment. While there are tremendous gains in information and ecological authenticity, clearly this more visible and flexible setting raises confidentiality issues that need to be taken seriously. As is true in any setting, here the client owns the confidentiality and is free to disclose or not to disclose the nature or the content of the visit. If the client chooses not to disclose who the home-visiting therapist is, there may be moments of social awkwardness over the lack of introduction or introduction by name only with no explanation. The client may also choose to introduce the therapist as a friend, a visitor, or as "someone from the county who is helping me now." Obvious limitations to confidentiality should be acknowledged and discussed with the client. These may include open windows with the neighbors working in the garden next door, family members in the next room, or inquisitive neighbors in a congregate living situation who may know the therapist on sight. In general, we have found that clients are not greatly concerned about these types of problems, but professional ethics requires that the therapist verify this in each case.

The change to the client's home will generally create a different social environment and requires some basic social ease and politeness on the therapist's part. However, this politeness should not disable the interviewer in conducting an assessment. While a bit more tact and diplomacy may be required in introducing delicate subjects, nothing that can be asked in an office cannot be asked at home. The therapist can maintain the same degree of control over content and pacing and ending the interview as at the office. With especially isolated and lonely clients, it can be very helpful to give a warning of the end of the visit, such as "I'm going to have to leave in about ten minutes. Is there anything else we should talk about?"

Since many people seem to consider the home visit client as captive to the interview, it should be pointed out that clients can and do cancel home visits or "fail to show" for appointments by not answering the door or leaving the house when the appointment is scheduled. Invitations to leave a client's home must be respected as well.

CASE EXAMPLES

The following examples taken from Senior Outreach practice serve to illustrate some of the assessment issues that can arise in outreach mental health team experience.

Dementia Versus Depression

Fred was a verbal, intelligent man in his early sixties who had retired from self-employment in an artistic field due to difficulty coming up with new ideas. His wife complained that he was not the same person, but when asked for specifics, she only noted his lack of interest in socializing or doing much besides sitting in his chair. Fred complained of lack of motivation. He had lost a few pounds and said he had trouble sleeping. He also complained of memory problems but gave no concrete examples. He did not appear depressed in mood, but he was not happy either. Mental status testing produced no errors except on delayed recall. Therapy for depression was started, and Fred developed a good relationship with the therapist and seemed to recall what was discussed from session to session. After a few months, he began to show up on the wrong day for appointments and walked home from a doctor's visit one day having been unable to find his car. Repeated mental status assessment showed no change, but further discussion of his reasons for avoiding social interaction suggested that it was too demanding for him to try to converse with former colleagues who understood his line of work. Joint sessions with his wife resulted in less pressure from her to socialize and also in her questioning some old acquaintances who told her for the first time of decline in the quality of his work prior to retirement. Therapy was terminated with support offered to the wife. Two years later she came forward after a community education talk to confirm severe progressive decline.

This case provides a good example of a highly educated, creative person for whom mental status testing yielded an inaccurate diagnosis of absence of cognitive impairment. Furthermore, his behavior was consistent with depression. In this instance, however, the withdrawal from social activity was his strategy for avoiding situations that were too complex for him. His weight loss was due more to forgetting to eat frequently than to lack of appetite. If he had been accurately diagnosed from the beginning, the intervention would have focused on the wife and would probably have been more efficient. Fred was able to benefit from therapy sessions in the first few weeks, but soon deteriorated to a level that made any lasting benefit unlikely.

Delirium Versus Depression and Dementia

David was in his seventies and barely responsive in the interview. His answers to mental status questions were inaccurate. His affect was flat to moderately depressed. His wife reported that he had lost thirty pounds over the past year and was sleeping a great deal. He moved quite slowly. He was taking an opiate-based pain medication for a progressive arthritic condition that he had suffered from for years. The team psychologist and psychiatrist who performed the initial assessment agreed that he was moderately to severely demented on the basis of mental status scores and other interview information but felt that he might also be depressed and that a trial on anti-depressant medication was worthwhile to see if his overall functioning would improve. The wife, who also was very emotionally distressed, was offered psychotherapy and accepted. The psychiatrist consulted with the primary care physician, and it was agreed to discontinue the opiates and to start anti-depressant medication. David's mood not only improved but his cognitive functioning increased tremendously to a level that his wife endorsed as normal. The "pseudodementia" appeared to be due to the pain medication and perhaps was exacerbated by depression.

David's case illustrates the opposite type of error in the sense that the mental status exam, even while used by experienced geriatric mental health professionals, identified David's cognitive impairment. Nothing about his behavior or history suggested an acute disorder. There were sufficient signs of depression that active psychiatric treatment was initiated. This treatment trial then serendipitously led to discontinuance of the opiate and recovery of functioning. This case suggests the degree of caution that must be used in diagnosis with the elderly, underscores the importance of attention to medication effects, and illustrates the ongoing nature of assessment and the use of treatment trials to clarify the diagnosis.

Bipolar Disorder Versus Dementia

Annie was interviewed in her home, which was disorderly and dirty. She was seated in a chair in the front room and dressed in clothes whose size suggested she had lost considerable weight although she claimed to be eating well. She failed to respond to most mental status questions and answered incorrectly when she did respond. Her speech was vague and digressive. The team members interviewing, both with several years of geriatric mental health experience, were uncertain whether she was demented or depressed or both. They did conclude that her functional status was sufficiently impaired that she needed to be hospitalized or placed in residential care. With considerable prompting, she produced from a notebook a written phone number that belonged to "a family member, I don't know who." A phone call proved this was her son in another town, who was shocked to hear of her current state. Discussion with him revealed that about a year previously she had had what sounded like a manic episode. With assistance from the son, who flew in to town the next day, she was moved to residential care and started on

appropriate medication. Her condition improved considerably, although she continued to suffer mood swings for several years, with
the depressions always characterized by severe cognitive impairment
that would remit as her mood elevated.

In this case, it is important to note that even though the diagnosis was
unclear, the functional impairment determined a course of action that also
led to further assessment. This example also illustrates the importance of
obtaining more history from family to better understand the current symptoms. While new cases of bipolar disorder are not common in late life, they
do occcur. Our experience in Ventura is that they are often accompanied
by cognitive impairment during the depressive phase. In any event, Annie
also demonstrated the presence of severe cognitive impairment due to
depression.

Dementia Versus Psychosis

Fran was referred to the team by the housing eligibility worker
because of deterioration in housekeeping, personal hygiene, and appearance. She was also described as confused. On the home visit,
team members saw that the house was sloppy and disorganized and
that she had not bathed in some time. Her make-up was garish, and
her clothes mismatched. She did poorly on mental status questions
related to place and time and reported having forgotten some things
about her own past. She felt someone might be stealing from her. In
some ways, she interviewed like a "typical" dementia case. However,
some of her mannerisms (e.g., the way she held her cigarette)
reminded one interviewer of institutionalized mental patients. When
the interviewer asked who the current president was, she volunteered that she did not know the previous one either. One team
member laughed and said, "You've answered these questions before,
haven't you?" This changed the tone of the interview and led to her
admitting that she had talked to psychiatrists before and had been in
state hospitals a large part of her life. After further discussion of this
history, we compared names to see if we knew some of the same
people at the nearest state hospital. She then went on to describe her
current problems as having the same symptoms as previous psychotic
episodes, including auditory hallucinations and suspiciousness of others and confused thoughts. A discussion of previous experience with

medication moved to negotiation about types and dosages that she would agree to take. She also felt that therapy had been helpful before, and a psychotherapist was assigned to provide a consistent relationship, reality testing, and some counseling in stress-coping skills. In a few months, the eligibility worker reported improved functioning, although Fran still reported some thought disorder.

Fran illustrates the importance of behavioral cues as an adjunct to the mental status exam. Except for the behaviors that suggested a history of institutional care, Fran might have been seen as demented. With this information, and the appropriate rapport, she supplied all the information that was needed for both diagnosis and treatment planning. The example also illustrates that mental status exams alone do not readily discriminate between dementia and schizophrenia which involves thought disorder and cognitive impairment.

Depression and Dementia

Clara was "going on eighty" and came in with complaints of memory loss and fear of getting "Alzenheimer's disease." Her complaints sounded to the interviewer more like cognitive slowing and concentration failures. She took longer to remember words and names, and she sometimes had to reread the beginning of a newspaper article because her attention wandered. She did well on the mental status exam. She also looked and acted sad and depressed. Further questions revealed a loss of interest in usual activities and a pervasive sense of life as "hopeless" and herself as "helpless and worthless." While not suicidal, she wished every day that "the Lord would take me in my sleep." Medication for depression was counterindicated for medical reasons. Fourteen sessions of psychotherapy improved her mood and eliminated her concerns about her memory.

The assessment illustrated in this example is relatively straightforward. It does, however, point to the importance of not taking memory complaint and self-diagnosis at face value. It also points to the need to be able to distinguish between concentration disorders, typical of depression, and true memory failure.

Depression and Illness

Agnes presented complaints of depression and a recent life history that suggested the typical losses that precede depression in late life: she had moved and did not like the new town, one friend had died, others had moved away. She felt tired and had no motivation to do things. Some days she would lie in bed all day. After five or six sessions, the therapist felt that Agnes did not really feel depressed nor was she acting in therapy like a typical depressed person. In fact, the only consistent complaint that remained after the first sessions was tiredness. The therapist recommended another visit to her primary care physician (whom she had seen regularly) to evaluate this tiredness. The physical exam and blood work revealed anemia; iron supplements cured the tiredness and the "depression."

In this instance, the lesson is that depression has a distinctive character and that its absence can be recognized even when one symptom (fatigue) and a typical life history is given. It also illustrates the important role that mental health can have in "ruling out" psychological explanations and referring for further physical evaluation.

Depression and Illness, Again

Susan was quite ill, having had two surgeries within a few months. At one point, she had been near death. Now, several months later, she was referred by her physician, who felt there was no physical reason for her to be housebound, in bed most of the time, and complaining of weakness. She made excessive phone calls to the doctor and had a number of emergency room visits with negative diagnostic results. The home visit assessment revealed numerous signs of depression and of panic disorder as well as a complex interaction with her husband, her primary caregiver, which was characterized by intense dependency on both sides and by hostility and guilt on hers. A fairly lengthy therapy involving both individual sessions and sessions for the couple resulted in an improved (though far from ideal) marital relationship, improved (if still frail) functional ability, a shift of phone calls from the physician's to the therapist's office, and in more appropriate use of medical services. Since she continued to be physically ill, regular communication with the physician was essential so that the therapist did not miss actual acute worsening of her medical condition, which did, in fact, occur twice during the psychotherapy.

This example shows the complex of physical problems, multiple psychological problems (depression, panic disorder, dependent personality), and marital problems that can occur in later life. It also serves as an important reminder that the physical/psychological question often results in a "both" answer rather than an "either/or."

SUMMARY

These few examples give some idea of the complexity and the challenge of assessment of older persons. The complexity arises both from determining the type of services needed (medical, mental health, social) and from the difficulty of differential diagnosis at this age. Diagnosis is more complex with the older adult and requires constant checking of the working hypothesis about the diagnosis. It is simply unrealistic to expect to be right all the time when working with older adults. What is essential is to be able to discover one's mistakes.

Diagnosis is the beginning of the therapeutic process, guides the choices of treatment strategies, and is informed by what happens in therapy. The next chapter offers a general description of therapy with the elderly and the differences and similarities between this kind of therapy and therapy with other populations.

RESOURCES

Readers interested in more information about assessment with the elderly are directed to the following books:

Zarit, S. H. *Aging and Mental Disorders.* New York: Free Press, 1980. The most thorough discussion of this area.

Birren, J. E., and K. W. Schaie, eds. *Handbook of the Psychology of Aging.* New York: Van Nostrand, 1985. Several chapters touch on assessment issues. The chapter by LaRue, Dessonville, and Jarvik is especially good.

Birren, J. E., and R. B. Sloane, eds. *Handbook of Mental Health and Aging.* Englewood Cliffs, N.J.: Prentice-Hall, 1980. Several excellent chapters on psychopathology.

Post, F. *Principles of Psychiatry in Late Life.* Oxford: Pergamon, 1965. Although more than two decades old, still a useful introduction. British psychiatry has been considerably ahead in recognizing and diagnosing psychosis in late life.

Reisberg, B. *Brain Failure.* New York: Free Press, 1981. Although dated by more recent advances, it remains a good introduction to Alzheimer's disease.

4

Therapy with the Elderly

Therapy with the elderly has been a topic of discussion in the professional literature for a number of years (see Rechtschaffen 1959; Kastenbaum 1964; Zarit 1980; Gatz et al. 1985; Knight 1986a, 1978–1979). While virtually all these discussions are optimistic in tone, the notion that older people are difficult, or at least different, in therapy still predominates. It is beyond the range of this chapter to provide a comprehensive description of therapy with the elderly or an analysis of the ways in which psychotherapy may need to be adapted to work with an older population of clients. My earlier work (1986) and the sources referred to therein can be consulted by readers who want more general information on the topic.

This chapter focuses on those aspects of therapy that require some adaptation to bring psychotherapists and older clients together and to clarify the role of psychotherapy within the outreach team context. My discussion therefore highlights the following issues: building rapport with older clients; the application of gerontological expertise in psychotherapy with older adults; how to use general therapy skills with the older adult population; the therapist's adjustment to illness, disability, and death as common issues in therapy; and special issues that arise in home visit psychotherapy.

BUILDING RAPPORT WITH OLDER CLIENTS

The initial contact with any potential client is, of course, critical to determining whether or not the therapy takes place at all. Older clients are both less likely to have defined their problems as psychological in nature (Gurin, Veroff, and Feld 1960; Knight 1986a, 1983) and to be presold on the value of psychotherapy as it relates to their problems. For these reasons, the initial contact (either the initial interview or even pre-interview telephone contacts to set up appointments) are usually more explicitly educational than is often necessary with younger adults who have grown up more familiar with psychotherapy.

The two questions to be addressed are: "Why is my problem a psychological one?" and "What will psychotherapy do for me?" Older people are more likely to conceptualize problems in somatic terms or as unsolvable life problems and less likely to diagnose themselves as depressed, anxious, and phobic and to seek help. Some careful explanation of how the problem could be seen in psychological terms is often necessary in order to engage the client's cooperation in the first interview.

Even given a mutual agreement on the problem or a willingness to consider the psychological explanation as a working hypothesis, the older person may still doubt that therapy can resolve the problem. Some explanation of the general ingredients of the therapeutic process is helpful: goal setting, the probable course of therapy, the benefit of talking to a skilled listener, and the value of expressing feelings. In addition, explanation in jargon-free terms of the therapist's conception of the value of therapy to this individual is also essential to engaging the older person in therapy.

This process is not without impact on the therapist. Many therapists practice with relatively little awareness of the decision-making process that clients go through before the first visit. For most clients consulting a psychotherapist, education about the therapeutic process takes place before the first meeting and is mostly done by friends, family, and other referral sources. Aside from clients who cancel appointments or who fail to return after a few visits, there is little confrontation with the views of the unconvinced about the value of psychotherapy.

In doing outreach work with older people, one is always to some extent selling psychotherapy to an unconvinced audience that often asks candid questions. In addition, the necessity of explaining what one has to offer in common language forces the therapist to confront the credibility of therapeutic ideas. To tell a housebound, physically disabled, and impoverished older person with seemingly intractable problems that he or she will feel better by talking to you for an hour a week and expressing his or her feelings can have a sobering effect on the most committed psychotherapist. Needless to say, if the therapist is uncertain about the value of therapy or his or her personal competence, outreach work will bring out these doubts.

The following sample dialogue shows one way to introduce an explanation of psychotherapy.

Case Example: Explaining Therapy

THERAPIST: Well, it sounds to me like a lot of your problems could be due to depression.

CLIENT: You mean that the pain is all in my head? I think that's what the doctor thinks.

THERAPIST: You think that's why she sent me, right? [Patient nods.] She doesn't think the pain is imaginary and neither do I. You have good physical reasons to hurt. I think that at least some of the tiredness you've been feeling, the trouble sleeping, the fact that food doesn't taste good, that you don't enjoy going to church anymore, all of that could be due to depression. And you have good reasons to be depressed; a lot has happened to you in the past three years.

CLIENT: So it's not imaginary?

THERAPIST: Do you think you could make this up? [Client smiles ruefully.] Anyway, why would you want to?

CLIENT: So how did I get this way?

THERAPIST: From my perspective, that may not be as important as what's happening to keep you depressed. Certainly the deaths in your family had a big impact, and the limitations on you since your last surgery have eliminated things you used to enjoy; other things may come up as we talk more. But my main strategy would be to look for ways we can change what you do and the way you think in order to break the cycle of depression. [This explanation is specific to this therapist's cognitive-behavioral approach to depression; other system explanations can be substituted as appropriate.]

CLIENT: So talking to you is going to help?

THERAPIST: Talking about it helps to relieve the pressure. Expressing feelings helps. The main change will come from changing the way you think about your life and finally from things you'll do differently.

CLIENT: Like what?

THERAPIST: Honestly, right now I don't know; part of the therapy will be us finding the answer to that question together.

CLIENT: But you believe you can help me.

THERAPIST: I've helped a lot of people like you.

CLIENT: As old as me?

THERAPIST: Even older.

EXPLAINING YOUTHFULNESS

Another aspect of building rapport concerns the age of the therapist. Although probably most critical for therapists who are, or who look, quite young, this can remain a problem well into middle age when dealing with clients who have children the therapist's age or older. In general, a bias against youth is best perceived and dealt with as if the client had asked the question: "What do you have to offer me?" By offering some description of his or her training, experience, and convictions about the nature of the work to be done, the therapist can allay the concerns of all but the most age-bigoted among the elderly.

On a somewhat more subtle level, building rapport can require showing a comprehension of the life circumstances, developmental issues, and common family problems, as well as the subculture of the elderly and even local history to provide some assurance of common understanding between the therapist and client. These problems are similar to those that arise with adults who may have a problem with a therapist of the opposite sex. One wants some reassurance that the therapist is not going to work from biases assumed to be associated with his or her gender. Thus, a male therapist learns to convey appreciation of competency, a sense of options, and an avoidance of sexist attitudes in order to build rapport with female clients. The female therapist learns to convey some appreciation of male difficulties in comprehending women, to build confidence in ability to read feelings, and to avoid blaming the male client for relationship failures. Similarly, the younger therapist must convey some appreciation of experience and history, a sense of client strengths, and an avoidance of age stereotyping or of siding with others in the family constellation.

Case Example: Handling the Client's Age-Bias

CLIENT: How could someone as young as you are help me?

THERAPIST: Obviously, I'm younger than you, but I wonder why you think that'll be a problem in helping you get over your panic attacks?

CLIENT: You don't understand what it's like to be old.

THERAPIST: If you mean I don't have personal experience of being older, obviously that's true. Actually, one of the things I think I've learned from reading about growing older and working with a lot of older people is that growing older is pretty much a unique experience for each person, so you'd have to tell me what it means for you in any case. What I do know about, though, is how psychotherapy works and quite a bit about panic attacks and how people get over them; don't you think that would be helpful?

CLIENT: [showing surprised interest] You studied panic attacks?

THERAPIST: Yeah, it's one of the main things psychotherapists do.

THE NEED TO UNDERSTAND GERONTOLOGY

As in the preceding examples, the ability to project an understanding of problems of older people and an appropriate level of comprehension of the experience and value of being older depends in some measure on the confidence that the therapists actually feel in their comprehension of aging and late life. Since much therapeutic work involves demonstrating empathy for people of other life backgrounds and people with different problems than those the therapist has, this empathic understanding is certainly not alien to the work of psychotherapy. However, it does appear that many therapists find it more difficult to empathize with older individuals than with others. It may be that a client's age and experience may encourage the therapist to identify him or her with parents, teachers, or supervisors. This may inhibit the therapist from using the same skills that would be used to comprehend persons of another gender, say, or of different cultural background or work experience.

The rapidly developing field of gerontology has helped us to comprehend older people and the aging process. Gerontological expertise can aid the therapist in building rapport and in helping older people understand aging (Knight 1986a). While the field of gerontology is fairly dense with facts, the information is rapidly changing with new research. In any case, this portion of a chapter is far too small to adequately summarize the field. Each therapist will have to commit to regular reading and continuing education to keep up with new knowledge.

Another major resource for the therapist is principles in thinking about aging that are derived from gerontological methodology. The methodological issues of research gerontology pose questions that challenge common social conceptions about the nature of aging and of older people. This research asks questions such as: Are observed features of older people due to the aging process itself? Are these features or differences due to being a member of a specific generation or age cohort? Are these differences due to being a member of a social subgroup (one which our society often treats as a minority group)? How much of what the person experiences is due to aging and how much to a specific illness, psychological disorder, social disorder? Is this a new problem arising in late life or a long-term problem whose subject has grown old with it?

With each question, there are some findings and directions provided by gerontological research and scholarship. The aging process appears to bring some slowing of cognitive processing, some ill-defined changes in memory performance, a greater interrelationship between physical and psychological processes, and perhaps a greater introspectiveness. It does *not* necessarily bring illness, disability, brain damage, political conservatism, introversion, or hypochondriasis.

Cohort membership, the group to which one belongs because of one's birth year, appears quite important in determining who we are, what attitudes we hold, and many if not most of the differences popularly ascribed to the aging process. The differences are real; but they are just attributes of particular groups and not of the process of aging. Each generation has a unique place in the ever-changing development of society, values, morals, and the nature of personal relationships. The therapist will need to devote some time in comprehending older clients as persons from earlier times who have a different culture than those born in later times.

Being an older person in our society implies the changes of social status that go with retirement: post-retirement marriage, segregated living arrangements, age prejudice, and age-based social policy (i.e., Medicare regulations, Medicaid regulations for long term care, Older Americans' Act programs). These factors create a social environment that is different for older members of our society, and while some differences are good and enjoyable, others are onerous. The therapist needs some understanding of all of these.

The comprehension of problems as specific to illness rather than aging often suggests different resources for understanding and for coping even if the problems are still irreversible. Understanding a progressive visual loss, for example, as due to a specific disease process helps to open up avenues of understanding the illness; learning about research that may someday lead to a cure for others; limiting the generality of the loss (e.g., quite possibly only vision will be lost, whereas the attribution to aging brings to mind the Shakespearian "sans everything"); and suggests recourse to counselors for the blind, talking books, and rehabilitative aids for the blind (e.g., cards that guide the visually impaired while signing checks and crecit card slips).

The differentiation of problems as new in late life versus being of a more long-term nature is of importance in not missing or misunderstanding the nature of many issues. There is considerable focus on dementia of the Alzheimer's type as a problem of late life because it is usually a late onset disorder. Other problems that affect large numbers of older people, such as schizophrenia and retardation, are problems with which people grow old. There may still be age-specific changes in the disorders themselves or age-related changes in treatment brought about by greater prevalence of other illnesses or the existence of different placement opportunities once the client is old. Other problems can go either way. For example, depression may have different meaning and possibly different treatment approaches depending on whether the client is experiencing another episode of a life-long series of depressions or is becoming depressed for the first time late in life.

In closing this section, I wish to emphasize that what I suggest here are questions that guide the therapist in thinking about aging and older people. These questions are also of considerable use in guiding older people to think about the aging process and their own experiences with older people. Without other input, the attempts of older people to understand aging and each another will, like the attempts of psychotherapists without gerontological expertise, fall back on social stereotyping. The largest scale survey to date on age stereotyping demonstrated the extent to which the elderly share in that process themselves (Harris and Associates 1975).

HOW TO GENERALIZE THERAPY SKILLS

Much of what has been written so far about therapy with the elderly raises questions about needing special skills to get the elderly into therapy and special assessment skills, as well as more familiarity with age-specific referral sources, with content areas more likely to arise in late life, and with suggestions for making changes in the pacing of therapy. However, there is nothing to suggest that different skills or different therapeutic techniques are necessary with older people.

Much of the work of applying therapy to older people is in freeing up the use of therapeutic skills that are easily applied to younger adults. In consulting with therapists about problem cases involving an older client, time and again the dilemma is in fact that the therapist knows what interpretation or other intervention to use but feels inhibited in saying that to an older person or in asking an older person to do a certain type of behavioral assignment. The reason for this inhibition generally says more about the therapist than about the nature of older people or the aging process. The following three examples illustrate this process of freeing up inhibited skills.

Example 1: Inhibition of Diagnostic Skill

Standing in the nurses' station area of a psychiatric ward, the geriatric team member is discussing an older gentleman admitted a few days previously. The charge nurse, ordinarily quite adept at assessment, is expressing confusion about the behavior the elderly patient has displayed. At this point, the team member has read the chart and has watched the client from a distance for a while.

CONSULTANT: Suppose he wasn't old, and you knew what's in the chart, and you were watching him right now—what would you think?
CHARGE NURSE: What do you mean?
CONSULTANT: Look at him and imagine he's twenty years younger; give him brown hair. What do you see? [The patient is noticeably shaky as he lights a cigarette and puts his feet down rather carefully as he walks.]

CHARGE NURSE: [reluctantly] Well, if he were younger, I would think he was an alcoholic.

CONSULTANT: Let's check it out. [She was right.]

Example 2: Incorrect Perception of Difference

After a presentation on mental health and aging to a group of community mental health center therapists, a clinical social worker came forward to describe with some excitement that he had been puzzled for some time as to why an older couple (in their seventies) he was counseling were talking about divorce. His comment: "I kept thinking, 'Why would old people want to get divorced?' While you were talking, it came to me: they want to get divorced for the same reason everyone gets divorced. They're miserable together; they have been for over twenty-five years."

Example 3: Withholding Confrontation

SUPERVISOR: You're feeling like the therapy is stuck, like you're not getting anywhere?

THERAPIST: Yes, she's just not dealing with her husband's death. I don't think she feels ready to. She just avoids it. I just don't think she's ready for therapy.

SUPERVISOR: You've had this come up before, right? [Therapist looks uncertain.] With younger clients. [Therapist nods.] What would you usually do then?

THERAPIST: [reluctantly] Well, I'd confront them and explain that this was an important part of their depression and that we needed to focus on it to get somewhere in therapy.

SUPERVISOR: Why not do that?

THERAPIST: I guess I think she couldn't handle it. I think of her as too frail to confront.

SUPERVISOR: [surprised] Is she? I haven't heard anything from you to suggest that this woman is fragile. And you have a good relationship at this point, right?

THERAPIST: [after some thought] Yes, I guess you're right. I still feel reluctant to do it, but there's really no reason not to.

THERAPISTS' ADJUSTMENT TO ILLNESS, DISABILITY, AND DEATH

From the therapists' viewpoint, work with older adults is different primarily in terms of exposure to frequent cases of clients who suffer from physical illness and especially chronic illness, from disability with limited or no hope of recovery of functioning, and clients who die during the course of therapy. This exposure poses a number of problems for therapists with no training in these areas or with limited professional or personal experience that prepares them for this work.

Given our society's general withdrawal from persons who are ill and who fail to get well (Parsons 1958) and from the dying (Kubler-Ross 1969), therapists beginning to work with elderly individuals may have their first personal experiences with these more or less taboo topics while doing therapeutic work. This first contact with harsher realities of life can produce considerable emotional shock and can lead to depression for the therapist and quite possibly to a desire to avoid this type of client. If the therapist is committed to such societal notions as hard work always pays off, serious illness can be avoided, and life is fair, these negative reactions will be still stronger. The problem is that chronic illness, the retirement practices of some employers, and the death of loved ones prior to long-planned pleasures in late life are more clearly and devastatingly unfair than the usual experiences of "unfairness" of those in their younger adult years.

The reactions of therapists can be intensified by the fact of their being "off time" in the sense of Neugarten and Hagestad's (1976) age-graded roles. That is, confronting chronic illness, disability, and death tends to be a normative task of middle age, frequently in the context of coping with one's parents' physical limitations and death. It comes ahead of schedule for the younger therapist working with older clients. It can also be problematic for the middle-aged therapist to confront the issues both at work and at home, since this violates the distancing between clinical and personal realities that enables many therapists to function effectively. Older therapists may have these issues resolved in their own lives but be inclined to want others to resolve these problems in the same way.

To some extent, many therapists protect themselves from the anxiety aroused by a client's problems by the recognition that they have handled this part of their life much better or at least differently than the client did. Working with clients who represent the therapist's future rather than past or present means that the therapist is constantly confronted with possible futures that cannot, in fact, be defended against by reference to one's own competence. Will I become disabled in late life? How good will my pension plan be after twenty years of inflation post-retirement? Will I become demented? Will I die? These questions, ignored by most Americans until events force them upon us, constantly confront the therapist working with older adults.

These issues often tend to be outside of typical training for psychotherapy, which is focused (as is most professional training) on younger persons with more acute and presumably more solvable problems. In fact, most psychotherapists, after paying lip service to not ruling out physical causes of problems, work on issues and with tools that are purely in the realm of thoughts and feelings. Working with individuals having very real and quite possibly irreversible physical limitations and injuries challenges the psychotherapist to confront realities that do not vanish in the face of confrontations of unconscious assumptions, emotional ventilation, restructured cognitions, changed reinforcement contingencies, insight, or other elements of the psychological armamentarium. These are not age-specific issues; younger adults do, of course, become disabled and die. But it is possible to work with younger adults and avoid these issues whereas it is not possible to work with older adults and avoid them. These psychological techniques are still valid, but they must be adapted to given realities and known abilities and disabilities.

Work with older adults confronts the clinician with the different experiences of clients who know themselves, know about the world, and know about relationships and who have run aground on issues that none of us handle very well and some that may not be handled but rather adapted to. Most therapeutic training prepares the clinician to (depending on the training metaphor) reparent, reprogram, or enable clients to relearn about themselves and so to correct faulty information gained from parents and childhood socialization experiences, with clients who are still learning about themselves and are relatively untested in the area of the psychological difficulty. Such change in clients may require various changes in the therapist: helping clients rediscover abilities rather than discover them for the first time; enabling clients to use areas of strength that the clinician may not have (more mature comprehensions of relationships, more courage in the face of death); and recognizing that some parts of life's difficulties are unfair and unsolvable.

The path to adjustment to these realities of work with the elderly are varied and incomplete. Some knowledge of gerontology and a broad experience with older people that includes those who are doing quite well in addition to those with problems can help prevent a sense of total despair and a feeling that all aging brings depression, disability, and dementia. The interdisciplinary team, when it actually functions as a team, can insulate against loneliness in the face of this sometimes difficult work. Training that emphasizes relevant and clinically enabling models of working with older adults prevents the unnecessary loss of clinicians who, sent to do work with older adults with tools and theoretical models that are suitable for work with adolescents and young adults, find themselves defeated by the experience of working with the aged. Clinical training must include some sensitive supervision that can explore the personal impact of this difficult work on the therapist. Finally, some people simply cannot function in this area because they do not have what it takes to work in the latter part of life.

THERAPY AND THE HOME VISIT

The effect of the home visit in altering the context of the initial assessment visit was covered in the preceding chapter. The home visit context can alter the nature of therapy in some ways, although in principle, there is nothing that can be done in an office setting that cannot also be done at home. The major challenge for the therapist is keeping the nature of therapy and the definition of the therapist's role clear in a setting that can encourage the client to confuse the therapist with other persons who come to the home to visit (home health nurses, friends, caseworkers) as opposed to people whom the client goes to an office to visit (physicians, clergy, teachers). The actual work of dealing with such distortions of the therapeutic alliance is similar for both settings, but because the roles with which the therapist is confused are different and because the ones associated with the home visit are often considered to be of lower status, the therapist may be confused or even insulted by transference reactions that would be handled naturally in an office context. From this viewpoint, there is no difference between explaining in the client's home that the therapist may not intervene to help the client get meals sent to the house or assist with applications for housing (as a caseworker would) or that the therapy will end someday and is not a relationship of mutual sharing of problems nor does it involve much purely social conversation or interaction (like friendship) and explaining in the office that the therapist is not offering immediately tangible solutions and answers (like a physician) or guidance in making value judgments and choices (as a pastoral counselor might).

This problem can intensify if the therapists themselves are uncertain of the role differences and have doubts about the definition and the value of psychotherapy. Seeing clients in their homes and without the comforting professional credibility of the office environment strips the therapeutic enterprise to its bare essentials: two people in a conversation designed to relieve one of them of problems—a process for which the other receives a fee.

One of the most common arguments against seeing clients in their own homes is that it increases the client's dependency on the therapist. Presumably, the therapist's expending additional effort and meeting the client on his or her home ground can evoke a transferential dependency that is much greater in magnitude than those generally observed in office-based practice. This, however, has not been our experience in eight years of home delivered psychotherapy. While some clients become dependent, their dependency does not appear to be related to the locale of the therapy. Clients seen in home situations are often more physically dependent due to an ongoing functional disability that precluded their coming to the office in the first place; one assumes that an experienced therapist knows and that a therapist in training can learn to distinguish between physical limitations and transferential dependency. A large part of this training may have to do with handling one's own countertransference concerning physical disability.

The perception of the locus of power in the relationship may differ depending on the location. Therapists often feel (perhaps not always realistically) that they are in control of the therapy when it takes place in their office. This sense of control is attenuated when therapy moves to the client's home, where the therapist is in the client's territory. In one sense, the therapist is always in control in that he or she guides the course of each therapeutic conversation and also guides the overall strategy of therapy. Yet, in another sense, clients always control therapy in that they decide what to incorporate into their daily lives and what to ignore for now as well as whether to return for the next visit. Neither of these viewpoints on who is in charge is dependent on the setting.

As was noted in the section on assessment in chapter 3, the therapist in the home setting may have to be more flexible in handling interruptions such as phone calls and unexpected guests as well as in seizing opportunities to spontaneously incorporate family members into therapy sessions. The development of ease in doing this is largely a training matter that can take place in school or on the job.

SUMMARY

In general, the argument presented here is that the major changes in providing therapy to the elderly lie in changes in the therapist's perception of therapy and of his or her role as a mental health professional. While technique may not change, there are significant changes in content and in the types of problems that the therapist may face in clients and the reactions these problems may evoke in the therapist. In a similar manner, the change to home delivery of therapy evokes a variety of personal reactions in the psychotherapist who has not been prepared by professional training for home visits. These changes present challenges for those who train therapists to work with the elderly whether on the job or in professional training programs.

The next chapter returns to the question of how to do effective outreach and bring referrals in so that the outreach team can provide assessment and active therapy to older adults.

5

Increasing Acceptance of Mental Health Services at the Community Level

Given the historical neglect of the elderly by outpatient mental health services and the widespread perception that mental health services have nothing to offer older people except assessment and inpatient treatment, education of potential clients and potential referral sources becomes an important strategy of outreach to older persons. Previous chapters have emphasized the importance of educating individual older clients about psychological disorders and the nature and function of psychotherapy. The lack of knowledge and the misperceptions regarding mental health and aging are so pervasive that strategies are needed to educate the community as well as individuals or families.

In general, there are four tasks that must be accomplished in order to establish the credibility of the outreach service in the local community. First, outreach team members must become known in the communities they serve. The second and third are essentially the same as with individual clients: the nature and presentation of psychological problems in older adults must be explained and the value of psychotherapy and psychotropic medication in working with these problems must be presented. Finally, good working relationships need to be established with the other agencies that comprise the local network of services to older people.

In small to moderate size communities, outreach does work, and people come to know and accept the mental health program for the aged as part of the community scene. This acceptance will likely reduce the need for outreach. But outreach will never discontinue since the scene of service agencies for the elderly constantly changes and since agencies experience relatively high turnover rates.

PERSONAL CONTACT WITH TEAM MEMBERS

While the stigma against mental health services is usually conceptualized at a rather abstract level, in day-to-day life experience it often comes down to prejudice against mental health professionals who may be perceived as anything from frightening to nice but irrelevant. Years of outreach experience suggests that this personal element is even more important in work with older people than it is with younger clients. In our society, younger people are somewhat more accustomed to seeking out mental health interventions and assessing the expertise of mental health professionals by their training, licensure, and other formal mechanisms. With older people, the perception appears to be the more concrete "this person can be of help" rather than the more abstract "I need a psychologist." Certainly, referral sources in the aging network find it easier to say, "I think Bob Knight could help with this depression you're having," rather than "You need to see a psychologist."

While conceptually simple, this need for personal exposure of the clinical team implies activities that do not come easily to many professionals and for which many mental health professionals have neither the training nor much inclination. It is necessary to develop skills in public speaking as well as teaching and to be able to relate well to a large variety of audiences. One is often called upon to justify (or even to sell) psychological concepts to audiences that are often neutral at best or at other times even hostile to the field of psychology. In addition, there is the need to be able to relate psychological concepts in jargon-free terms.

These skills are fairly easy to learn. However, very few training programs for therapists provide training in public speaking or in the presentation of psychological concepts to lay audiences. In fact, many programs seem to encourage their students to view these practices as outside of the professional role of the practicing therapist.

EXPLAINING PSYCHOLOGICAL PROBLEMS

As with the older client seen on an individual basis, the goal of community education about psychological disorders is to increase understanding of these problems and to assit the audience in recognizing such disorders in themselves and in others. Since most audience members, unlike clients, are not suffering from such disorders and may not have symptoms or other problems to which the talk can directly relate, the presentation will have to be more general in nature. It will also be necessary to relate the material to signs of such problems that the audience may see in others, since in many cases the people who attend the talks will not be potential clients themselves but will know of others who may be.

One common danger in such presentations is that mental health workers will try to communicate this information as if they were speaking to their colleagues. It is important to consider the audience's point of view. It is unlikely that the audience will have much information about categories of psychological disorders or that potential clients will have disclosed the type of personal and detailed information with which a diagnosis is determined. Whether aimed at community elderly or at workers in aging service centers, one goal of such talks is to help the audience to recognize possible referrals; it is not to enable them to actually diagnose clients.

In fact, if clients' peers or even other service providers learn to recognize some types of mental disorder that they may now dismiss as normal aging or eccentricity, this may well have negative consequences for the client. For example, whereas it is of some importance that family members who are caregivers understand the nature of Alzheimer's disease, some workers in long-term care settings in certain regions identify Alzheimer's disease with a tendency to persistent wandering and aggressive behavior. This different perception can lead to family members inadvertently narrowing their choices in long-term care by having staff incorrectly identify the patient as a problem patient when the individual may be like the majority of the patients in the facility. In the same sense, the integration of older schizophrenics in the community may depend on the misperception that they are "just old" and therefore eccentric or even that they have dementia rather than psychosis.

Another goal of such talks is to communicate clearly that having a need for mental health services is not equivalent to being crazy or psychotic. It is important to indicate the kinds of problems that can be addressed in outpatient mental health—problems that range from relatively normal problems in coping with unusual levels of stress in one's life through intense emotional reactions like depression. It is also of importance to distinguish other problems from Alzheimer's disease, both in terms of the essential differences in the problems themselves and in terms of the greater hope for positive outcome in treatment of adjustment disorders, depression, anxiety states, and so forth.

The therapist will have to decide at what level to provide information. If one is just beginning to speak to community groups, it is likely that one will want to cast the net relatively widely and to sort out the true cases from among others incorrectly identified as needing help. As time goes on, it will be possible to narrow the process somewhat, but some allowance will always be needed for difference in perception between trained diagnosticians and community persons who want to be of help. Whereas one may eventually want to give guidance in separating the clinically depressed from the merely "sad and blue" in terms of intensity and duration of the depressed mood, the assessment of suicidality is probably best left to the professional. Similarly, while it may be possible to communicate that not everyone who is forgetful is depressed and so in need of referral, it will not be possible to have referral sources distinguish between demented people who are socially withdrawn and those who have a depression superimposed on dementia and those who have depression with some cognitive impairment as a symptom.

Depending on the current sophistication of the community in which the team will operate, the topics of educational subjects programs may need to begin with relatively non-threatening topics such as discussions of sleeping problems, getting along with others, making friends, or adapting to the death of a husband or wife. Alzheimer's disease and depression are becoming recognized in the community of elderly as are other issues that relate to psychological problems. The concepts of stress and stress-induced or stress-exacerbated illness are also good transitional topics to discussions of psychological problems. Anxiety, phobias, and the nature of psychotherapy tend to be rather threatening and therefore should be explored only in groups with relatively sophisticated knowledge. Discussions of psychosis and of keeping the long-term mentally ill in the community are quite possibly taboo. Series of talks on grieving, coping with stress, coping with memory changes in late life, and communicating clearly can also be good topics through which outreach team staff can be introduced to the community. These lecture/discussion series can evolve into more personal discussions of individual problems, including observations on how therapy might help.

DEMYSTIFYING PSYCHOTHERAPY

For the majority of older people, psychotherapy is a relatively recent development within their adult lives. People who have grown up and been educated since psychotherapy has become accepted and openly discussed socially as well as in the arts and media may have difficulty appreciating how new the concept is for people who were middle aged when therapy became widely available and gained some degree of acceptance. Many older people equate mental health with long-term inpatient hospitalization of people who were thought disordered or bizarre in action. This is more common among the elderly who lived outside of metropolitan areas or who were not wealthy enough to afford or to be exposed to those engaged in lengthy psychoanalysis, the most common form of therapy prior to the 1950s.

The basis of teaching prospective clients about psychotherapy is described by Orne and Wender (1968) and evaluated as successful with a variety of groups by Garfield (1978). Often described as the role induction method (borrowing from hypnotherapy the idea that clients need to be "inducted" into the client role), it involves teaching these points: one does not have to be mentally ill to benefit from therapy; talking to a trained listener brings relief; goals are set by the therapist and client together; a description of the scheduling and timing of therapy for the client's presenting problem; and a discussion of the fees likely to be involved.

This process can be of great value in work with older people and as a guideline for community education talks on therapy to older adults, to other workers in the network of services for the elderly, and in other settings such as discussion groups, senior health fairs, and family support groups. It is important neither to oversell nor to undersell the benefits of mental health services. Psychotherapy is probably about as useful as casework, education, or health services; it is certainly not a panacea for the problems of aging.

TALKS ON AGING

For the mental health professional trained in gerontology, a major method for explaining psychological problems, demystifying therapy, and gaining personal exposure in the community is talks on aging. These talks may be addressed to older people themselves, to younger adults as family members of the elderly, or to professionals and service providers of varying levels of training and familiarity with the topic. There are a variety of topics that can be useful in such talks.

Normal Aging

Often presented as demythologizing late life, this topic is a favorite of gerontologists and especially of people relatively new to practice in the area. It can be very useful as an introduction and to establish credibility. One should avoid discussing it repeatedly because the lessons that can be drawn from gerontology at present are fairly simple and easy to learn and the audience is likely to retain the information from one talk to the next. In general, this topic should be avoided with groups familiar with the elderly unless one is certain that one has new and surprising information.

Alzheimer's and Other Dementias

These topics are currently of great interest and often draw good attendance and inspire questions during discussion. There is considerable information available on the topic in the general media and one should have more expertise to speak on Alzheimer's disease. Strategically, it is of considerable importance to contrast treatable and untreatable dementias with one another and with depression and changes due to normal aging. It is a disservice to older adults if the audience leaves fearing that they have Alzheimer's disease because they misplace their car keys from time to time.

Coping with Stress

Stress and its relationship to disease are of considerable interest and importance to older adults, many of whom have physical disorders that were caused and/or are now exacerbated by stress. These talks can explore the relationship between illness and aging as well as consider common stressors of late life, such as disability, the loss of loved ones, changes in family roles, relocation, and so forth. The topic also lends itself to opening up areas of psychological intervention, including the need for behavior change in coping with stress and illness, the role of relaxation therapies of various kinds, and the role of counseling and psychotherapy in the treatment of physical illness.

Common Psychological Problems in Late Life

This discussion is a good intermediate or advanced topic for a group one has a relationship with. It is useful as a bridge between relatively common experiences, such as loneliness, grief, and normal sadness and worries, and more serious problems, such as depression, anxiety disorders, phobias, and paranoia.

Family Problems in Late Life

This topic is frequently used, but all too often by people who consider the topic to be limited to discussing their views on the appropriate time to institutionalize the older family member or to seek conservatorship. At a minimum, such talks should distinguish between families of normal older people, families of the physically frail, and families of cognitively-impaired elderly. Some acknowledgement of the complex histories and dynamics of older family systems and of the possible distortions in perceptions of older family members caused by old parent-child conflicts and by the middle-aged family members' fears of aging is also necessary to assure that the presentation does more good than harm.

Grieving

While not specific to late life, grieving is a common experience among elderly people and in some settings a talk on coping with grief can be very useful as an introduction to mental health concepts. Some discussion of the differences between grief and depression and of the role of support groups and therapy in coping with prolonged or unusually intense grieving can be very helpful.

Making Friends

Social psychology offers some guidelines on the nature of friendship and on the ways that people meet, interact, and grow close. Older people, drawing on a lifetime of experience, themselves have interesting ideas about what friendship means and how friends are made. Such talks can help people find new strategies for making friends, come to terms with decisions they are making not to work hard at making new friends, and appreciate the importance of having someone to confide in.

Clear Communication

Learning elements of communication, attending to nonverbal messages, and understanding the emotional meaning of messages can be interesting and useful to older adults. The examples that the audience brings up often provide a transition to future topics in family issues and stresses of aging.

Assertive Training

This is often interesting and helpful to older adults, who may not, however, accept the values implicit in the assertive training package. In our geographical area (Ventura), it has often been helpful to call it something else (e.g., "Clear Communication II") since "assertive training" per se seems to have gotten a bad connotation among the elderly. But whatever it is called, this topic is helpful for introducing people to some of the assumptions and values implicit in psychotherapy.

Introduction to Diagnostic Groups

Usually aimed at people working with the elderly, this topic can acquaint these workers with the typical behavior of some types of psychological disorders. The presentation must be geared to the audience and be intended to increase understanding and acceptance of people rather than labeling and rejection of them. To this end, it is of great importance that the presenter know the context in which the worker encounters problems and what the worker must do with that person as well as be able to suggest concrete solutions to the worker's problem (which is usually the need to complete a specific task with someone who is either not comprehending the task or not attending to it because of emotional distraction). Such workers are not likely to need or desire a theoretical discourse on etiology or training in therapeutic listening skills. Job-related interventions are desired. Also, regardless of one's feelings about the medical model of psychological disorders, it is often more useful for people to conceive of the client as ill rather than as intentionally frustrating their attempt to do their job.

Community Service Discussion Group

As an adjunct to talks and to therapeutic services, discussion groups offered in sites where seniors gather can be a very useful outreach mode. These groups tend to vary between educational model lecture and discussion groups to meetings that are distinguished from group therapy mainly by a somewhat lower level of self-disclosure and confrontation. They can provide a convenient resource for the host agency to send people who may want therapy to meet the potential therapist; they can serve an ongoing educational function; and they can offer support for people who do not need therapy. These groups can also provide a useful entry point into recreation centers and meal sites for former clients who are looking for that type of community support.

NETWORKING WITH OTHER AGENCIES

The need to function as an integrated part of a larger network of services for clients is certainly not new to the field of community mental health nor to nurses and social workers. But physicians, psychologists, and other people whose training and work experience frequently involve large, complex and relatively self-sufficient hospitals and other institutions, may find the concept new and frightening. The complex needs of the older client will necessitate working with aging network service providers, social services, health care providers, the legal system, and so on. This need for interdisciplinary and inter-system cooperation requires both conceptual understanding of how systems should, can, and do work together and practical training in manipulating complex systems for the good of the client. Such an operational framework must include an understanding of the differences among what agencies say they do, how they operate on a day-to-day basis, and how they can sometimes be made to do things they do not usually do. Ideally, systems can be comprehended in such a way that identified problems can be resolved either by adjusting the system or by creating new services. An example of the geriatric's team role as a community change agent is laid out in some detail in the next chapter on dementia services.

The role as referral agent in the fuller sense of making accurate referrals that will provide the client with a service (as opposed to the limited but all too common sense of handing out phone numbers obtained from lists or pamphlets) is likely to have been part of the training of social workers or nurses on the team and should be learned and used by other team members as well. This role involves, for example, recommending that the family continue to provide certain transportation because local services only provide transport to medical visits. It may also involve letting the client know that his or her best options for reduced workload may be in getting assistance with housekeeping and with bathing where companion or friendly visiting are less available in a particular community. Knowledge about waiting lists for various services is essential in giving clients and families advice about planning ahead. Finally, for limited numbers of cases, special consideration may be obtained for given clients if equal flexibility is offerred in return. Examples of such flexibility for the mental health team may be the willingness to do a field evaluation on a referral of a case that does not sound at all like a mental health case or the willingness to change a schedule to see a case that appears to be an emergency to the referral source but not to the team.

Understanding the aging services system is useless, however, if the individual worker is not able to form good relationships with the other individuals who work in the system. In addition to basic social skills, developing such relationships requires some ability to take the other's point of view. While therapists do this constantly with clients, many seem unaware that the same skills are valuable in dealing with colleagues, especially those in other disciplines.

Discipline-specific training programs often inadvertently undermine such cooperation by encouraging the development of a positive professional self-image by denigrating other professions. Workers in the aging network need some positively toned understanding of other workers in other disciplines, including nurses, physicians, social workers, psychologists, attorneys, and the wide array of professionals and paraprofessionals who have an impact on the lives of older people. In principle, this training should include contact with trainees or practicing professionals from these other disciplines.

For the practicing professional, this understanding of the system is applied by recognizing and using opportunities to become acquainted on a more personal basis with the people who staff the local services to the elderly. Efforts to do so can include attending training meetings, serving on advisory boards, and going to open-house functions for services. They may also require broadening one's concept of expertise and the perception of one's own professional role: that is, interdisciplinary cooperation involves everyone's taking advice from those who may be "lower" on the traditionally defined hierarchy and everyone's doing things that may not be part of the usual job description or professional role.

In this sense, it should be common in the geriatric outreach setting to find all members listening intently to perspectives about clients offered by volunteers, nurses' aides, homemaker aides, and meal-site workers. They all offer valuable perspectives on the client who is being helped. In fact, the usual economies of health and social systems dictate that those with the least training and status will have the greatest actual exposure to the client and therefore the largest and best samples of behavioral observation (e.g., the client's physician sees him or her five to ten minutes a month, the home health nurse half an hour per month, the homemaker aide eight hours per week). By the same token, all team members will be doing information and referral, occasionally running errands for homebound clients (as time and relationship considerations permit), bringing bedbound clients glasses of water, checking refrigerators for food (and spoilage), and checking on compliance with medication by counting remaining pills.

In general, all workers in the aging network setting must accept that all of the others present in this setting are at their highest level of training and are competent to do their jobs. The level of egalitarianism must be rather high; otherwise, the mental health worker's assumption of higher status due to degree level or discipline is likely to neutralize his or her effectiveness in the community. Credibility in this setting must be earned by service to clients rather than bought with years of education. The complexity of the interacting problems of older people and their families is more than a textbook truism and the rather worn parable of the blind men and the elephant is an apt metaphor for interdisciplinary interactions as well as for the interaction of the service system with the family system. The achievement of true competency will come from understanding all of the interacting players, the willingness to get one's hands dirty with work not typically considered part of the office-bound, private-practice-model mental health professional role, and the easy acceptance of the expertise of other players on the team helping "your" client.

SUMMARY

This focus on outreach is best understood within the context of a particular application. The following chapter discusses services for the demented elderly and their families and also provides a context for viewing in more detail the integration of community education, the direct service provision of assessment and psychotherapy, the necessity of understanding and operating within a complex network of services, and the usefulness of community organization strategies to introduce a new supportive service elements, such as self-help groups for families of the demented, in the community.

RESOURCES FOR TALKS

There are a variety of texts and popular books that can be used to prepare talks for community groups. The following list of readings is intended to be suggestive rather than inclusive.

Alzheimer's Disease and Caregiving

Zarit, S. H. *Aging and Mental Disorders.* New York: Free Press, 1980. Good background on dementia, depression, and behavioral interventions for both.
Reisberg, B. *Brain Failure.* New York: Free Press: 1981. A good readable review of information on dementia and major theories of Alzheimer's disease.
Zarit, S., N. Orr, and J. Zarit. *The Hidden Victims of Alzheimer's Disease.* New York: New York University Press, 1985. A very readable description of the USC program for caregivers of memory-impaired elderly.

Death and Dying

Kubler-Ross, E. *Death and Dying.* New York: Macmillan, 1969. The classic work in this area. Presents good advice for the clinician and empathy for the dying patient.
Rando, T. *Dying, Death, and Grief.* Champaign, Ill.: Research Press, 1984. Rando makes clear the important distinction between adjusting to one's own death and to that of loved ones. A valuable resource with practical advice and the best literature review available.

Clear Communication

Gottman, J., et al. *A Guide to Couple's Communication.* Champaign, Ill.: Research Press, 1976. Designed to be used with couples, it has many exercises and examples that are useful in any class on communicating.

Assertive Training

Rimm, D. C. and J. C. Masters. *Behavior Therapy.* New York: Academic Press, 1974. Good resource for practice of several behavioral techniques.

Goldfried M. R. and G. Davison. *Clinical Behavior Therapy.* New York: Holt, 1976. Good discussion of assertion and the other techniques from a more cognitively-oriented perspective.

Depression

Lewinsohn, P. M., R. F. Munoz, M. A. Yougren, and A. M. Zeiss. *Control Your Depression.* Englewood Cliffs, N.J.: Prentice Hall, 1978. Designed to be used by members of depression classes. Many good exercises and course outlines.

Coping with Stress

Pelletier, K. *Mind as Healer, Mind as Slayer.* New York: Delta, 1977. A good overview of mind-body interaction in disease with discussion of relaxation, autogenic training and other methods.

Benson, H., and M. Z. Klipper. *The Relaxation Response.* New York: Avon Press, 1976. Develops the generalized concept of stress and the importance of relaxation in disrupting cycles of building stress.

6

Services for the
Demented Elderly

The demented elderly comprise a significant subgroup of older people with serious needs for services and support from the community. Dementing illnesses, principally dementia of the Alzheimer's type and multi-infarct dementia, increase in prevalence with each decade of life. There is a large proportion of demented elderly in the population of institutionalized older people. These two factors have led in the past to the erroneous identification of dementia as the only or at least the major mental health problem of the elderly. Aside from its inaccuracy (the elderly have a variety of mental health problems, the most prevalent of which is depression), this error has caused two types of problems. One is a general pessimism about mental health services for older people based on the assumption that most if not all are suffering from organically based and therefore untreatable mental disorders. The attempt to correct this earlier misperception has led to a second problem. The emphasis on the needs of the nonorganically ill population and education of the public and professional communities about other disorders has continued to ignore the needs of those with dementing illnesses.

In general, mental health professionals receive relatively little training about brain disorders. Usually, the array of mental disorders is divided into those with organic etiology and those with functional etiology. The primary focus of training thereafter is on the functional disorders. There is a strong, if usually implicit, assumption that functional disorders are treatable and organic ones are not. This bias tends to be preserved even in light of two recent developments that tend to blur the distinction itself as well as the assumption that treatability is determined by etiology. Two classically defined functional disorders (schizophrenia and bipolar affective disorder) are increasingly considered to be organic in origin. Both are also more usually considered to be managed rather than treated, whether through medication only or a mix of medical and psychosocial interventions. Nevertheless, these disorders are generally seen as clearly within the mental health services spectrum, whereas other organic disorders may be excluded. This exclusion is more perplexing when the same psychotropic medications may be used and the same psychosocial interventions may be implemented (casework, day care programs, and hospital milieu, among others).

The other recent development that makes the exclusion of the organic disorders questionable is the increasing role of psychological services (usually styled as health psychology or behavioral medicine) for disorders that were previously considered not only clearly "organic" but also not mental at all. Psychosocial interventions are often incorporated into the care of heart patients, cancer patients, diabetics, and others with long lasting physical disorders.

What is special about the dementing elderly? Those far along in the development of the dementing disorder lose language ability, memory, and other cognitive functioning to a degree that makes the practice of verbally based interventions like psychotherapy absurd. Since the very demented (and especially those who live together in institutional settings) are the best-known examples of demented elderly, much of our thinking and public policy is no doubt based on those who are, in this sense, beyond therapy. Even these individuals may benefit from psychotropic medication, behavioral interventions, and environmental modification. But dementing illness is, in general, progressive. A fundamental, and so far unanswered, question is this: At what point in the dementing process does the demented older person become so incapacitated as to no longer profit from psychotherapy? As we become better at early detection, an answer to this question will become essential. Even now, some older people in early stages of dementing illness and with an awareness of what is to come are being denied access to one source of assistance in coming to grips with a difficult and frightening reality in their lives.

Perhaps even more distressing is that in ignoring the needs of the demented elderly another and probably more needy group is also generally ignored: caregivers to the demented older person. The caregiver is often under more stress and suffers more emotional distress than does the demented person. Many, though certainly not all, are sufficiently distressed to have a DSM-IIIR classifiable disorder. Recent studies suggest that between 25% and 80% of caregivers may be clinically depressed (Fiore, Becker, and Coppel 1983; Rabins, Mace, and Lucas 1982; Cohen, personal communication, 1988). Given the strong identification of the victim of Alzheimer's disease as the patient, it can be difficult to get either the professional provider or the caregiver to perceive the need for the caregiver to be identified as the client and as the logical point of intervention into the complex needs of the caregiving family.

The following discussion describes the work of the Ventura Senior Outreach Team from 1980 to 1987 and suggests a potential model for mental health services for the demented elderly and their families. This model involves intervention at the community level, with families, with the principal caregiver, with the demented person, and with organizing caregivers into groups for mutual support and community action. The model and its rationale were directly copied from the education, support group, and individual counseling model developed by Steven Zarit and Associates at the Andrus Older Adult Center at the University of Southern California, described by Zarit (1980) and by Zarit, Orr, and Zarit (1985). The focus on an individualized, problem-solving model for coping with the behavior problems of the demented is useful in the community mental health setting in that it guides interventions at individual, group, and community education levels. Their university based program was adapted to the community mental health center setting and to some degree extended.

LEARNING ABOUT DEMENTIA

In order to be of assistance to dementing persons and their caregivers and families, one must, of course, know something about dementia. While this requirement would seem to be obvious, there are enough "instant experts" around sharing misinformation that a basic standard of knowledge needs to be described. At a minimum, one should know about the more common dementing illnesses, the reversible conditions that can mimic or cause temporary dementia, and the assessment procedures that can be helpful for diagnosis, including medical assessments and mental status assessments. An up-to-date knowledge of research in the field, including prevailing theories as to cause, progress toward better medical assessments, and the possibility of treatment, rehabilitation, or amelioration of symptoms, is essential when addressing groups in the community or working with families who are typically hungry for knowledge. It is equally important to be current on those possible treatments that are receiving media attention and to help families evaluate such reports.

A thorough knowledge of the caregiving process and the stresses attendant on being a full-time caregiver is also an essential part of the basic repertoire of knowledge that the service provider should have. A sense of how caregivers are selected, who they are, the dynamics of interaction in caregiving families, and the sources and remedies for caregiver stress as well as the probable consequences of ignoring caregiver burden is also important professional knowledge.

One also needs to be thoroughly aware of community resources for both home-based and institutional care. In providing such information to families, one must distinguish clearly between recommendations and unrated lists of available resources. In order not to create false hope, the professional needs to know what services are actually provided as well as being candid about what is not provided in the community. Far too many professionals and service agencies avoid telling people that there are no appropriate services by passing callers on to other agencies who pass them on to still others and keep the unending referral chain going.

In addition to knowledge, one needs experience with a wide variety of types of dementing illness, levels of dementing illness, settings in which the dementia occurs, caregivers, and family types and dynamics, and to be acquainted with the full range of services that provide assistance to the demented and their families, including those that may not be identified as specific to dementia or even realize they service the demented among others. All too many professional service providers have experience with the demented in only one type of setting and lack awareness of the selectivity of that setting. Listening to people who work in institutional care, in day care, in a medical school hospital, and in home health discuss demented elderly persons rather forceably brings to mind the parable of the blind men describing an elephant.

Finally, knowledge about dementia is new and rapidly changing. One must constantly give up old knowledge in the face of new. It is also wise to be careful about contradicting caregivers on the basis of textbook knowledge. Their experience is immediate and intense and needs explaining when it contradicts what ought to be true in terms of theoretical knowledge about the disease process, or else "what ought to be true" must be reconsidered. For example, while it used to be taught that dementia had an average course of six to ten years, we did groups for caregivers with fifteen to twenty years of in-home caregiving experience with the demented. On a different level, given a diagnosis of Alzheimer's disease, it can be helpful to lead families to reinterpret what they saw as a recent sudden onset as an unnoticed progressive decline, since they have often misinterpreted the patient's earlier behaviors in ways that carry emotionally charged meanings for some family members (e.g., "Dad didn't want me to know about that" becomes "Dad forgot about that and couldn't have told me"). Caregiver experience and research knowledge need to be complementary and interactive rather than oppositional.

COMMUNITY EDUCATION ABOUT DEMENTIA

In many communities, the mobile outreach team is the most expert group in disorders of late life, including the dementias. It is, in general, desirable to increase the sophistication of the community about dementing illnesses, especially concerning diagnosis and the range of possibilities for managing demented older persons at various stages of the illness. It is obviously of great importance that diagnosis be good enough that persons with reversible dementias are detected as early as possible and treated.

Yet education about dementia is not without unintended negative effects. For the community of elderly, frequent exposure to talks on dementia is likely to increase fears of having dementing illness and contribute to anxiety and depression. Increased focus on the possibility of memory loss and perceived changes in memory with age and the great difficulty of distinguishing between early-stage dementia and perceived benign memory changes create the possibility of education leading to constant apprehension and self-monitoring. Persons already moderately and clearly demented and particularly their families often deny their condition. For such people and their families an emphasis on accuracy in diagnosis that leads to repeated testing may do little except annoy and upset the patient and deplete the family's resources. Some sectors of the network of services for the elderly are quite open to serving people who are "simply old and forgetful", but perceive people with Alzheimer's disease as being unmanageable or always assaultive. Increasing the labelling of people as "demented" may thus unintentionally close off services that are currently available. The possibility of these unintended negative consequences must be weighed in planning talks and responding to audience questions.

In the first step of planning community education talks about dementia, one must therefore consider the likely audience (e.g., older people, social service workers, professionals in mental health, physicians, long term care workers), goals for the talk (increased knowledge, behavior change, policy change), and possible unintended consequences (Can the information lead to undesired effects for clients? Is there any way to prevent those effects or make them less likely?).

The audience makes a great deal of difference in the focus of the talk. A general talk directed to older people should largely focus on defining dementia, describing common causes, and emphasizing the recognition of common causes of reversible confusion (e.g., depression, malnutrition, medication problems, and endocrine imbalance, among others). In order to allay fears, the talk may emphasize common benign memory complaints and evidence that these do not usually progress to serious dementia. A talk directed to family caregivers, on the other hand, should emphasize the importance of accurate diagnosis and include some standards to indicate when a sufficient degree of certainty has been attained. Caregiver audiences will want to know about stress and stress management as well as locally available options for respite. Social service workers will be interested in assessment and respite options and may need to hear that Alzheimer's patients and those people whom they have been used to thinking of as "senile" or "simply old" are largely the same group under a different name. Physician audiences will need more diagnostic specificity and may need to be encouraged to take caregiver reports more seriously and to think of the caregiver as a patient as well as the demented person.

The goals of educational presentations in the community must be clearly thought out. Many presentors seem to expect that increased knowledge will lead to correct action and to needed changes in behavior or policy. In most cases, such changes are unlikely. If one is hoping for specific changes, the talk must spell out those changes and the rationale for them; one must also anticipate barriers to the audience acting on the new information. For example, any recommendation to spend more time with family caregivers must recognize the tremendous time pressure that physicians and long-term care staff experience. One can then argue that a little more time listening now will save time by preventing repeated phone calls and later confrontations that are stressful for everyone.

It must also be recognized that some families are under so much stress that referral to a professional counselor is indicated. If there is time for question and answer discussion, one can explain that while long-term-care staff often feel too busy to orient and educate families as to what to expect (which they can do and do quickly), they also feel responsible to handle complex emotional outbursts and family dilemmas which would better be referred to professional counselors and take up tremendous time and emotional energy.

Much of the change that is hoped for from educational talks requires longer involvement with the audience and necessitates a change from lecture style to case consultation, behavioral coaching, and intervention at management levels. Some desired change, such as staff's interacting more with individual patients, may simply be unrealistic given the economics of program budget and limited staff time. In short, education is helpful and can reach large groups of people with information, but it is limited in impact and unable to address problems that require more individual attention. No one has given up denial as a defense against the emotional strain of long-term caregiving just because a presentor said he or she should.

DIRECT SERVICES

Professional mental health services can interact with the dementing older person and his or her family in a variety of useful ways and can be an important part of the overall support network for that person. The logical points of interaction for the mental health professional with the demented person and the family are assessment, education, referral for other services, and therapy for the caregiver.

The specifics of assessment were covered in chapter 3. With regard to dementia, the mental health professional has an important contribution in establishing the presence of dementia by the evaluation of mental status for cognitive impairment and by ruling out other potential psychological disorders, such as depression, schizophrenia, or paranoia. Clearly, mental health assessment alone is never enough; medical evaluation is always needed to rule out possible acute medical factors. But mental health assessment is nearly always needed because very few non-psychiatrist physicians are good at complete mental status assessment or at distinguishing among mental disorders.

Assessment of the dementing older person continues to be important after initial diagnosis so that families can be assisted in understanding the progression of the illness and the patient's missing cognitive abilities and their consequences in day to day life as well as the patient's remaining abilities. Families are often slow to grasp the implications of memory loss; they often say, "Yes, I know Dad has Alzheimer's, but why does he forget where I've gone when I run to do an errand?" Understanding the complexity of mental functioning and its relationship to brain deterioration is a challenge even for brain researchers. Families need assistance in accepting some losses as real in the face of preserved ability in other areas.

A caregiver may say: "I think my husband is faking it for attention. He says he can't balance the checkbook, but I know he remembers all his old childhood stories." The error here derives from a prevalent misperception of memory as a unitary cognitive process that is either working or not. The professional consultant can be of help to both patient and family by assisting the family caregivers in comprehending the possibility of losing some memories and not others and of losing some cognitive functions and not others (e.g., being unable to retain new information, such as where the caregiver went and what time he or she will return, but being able to recall old material, such as who won the 1957 World Series.)

There is also the ongoing need for assessment of behavioral problems displayed by the dementing person. While there are typical and atypical behavioral problems, they occur in a complex context of cognitive misunderstanding by the patient, unintentional reinforcement by the environment, and family dynamics, all of which exacerbate the displayed problem. Understanding the problems, learning to change the behavior or adjust to it, and learning to change oneself and others in the family in order to accommodate the dementing older person represent the ongoing challenges of the caregiver for the dementing person. For example, considerable emotional tension, including aggression by the patient, may occur in a context in which the daughter and her husband are leaving while the demented father asks over and over where they are going. The daughter, feeling guilty about leaving and sensing (or projecting) her husband's impatience, keeps answering but gets more and more tense, a state that the father reflects and amplifies. A very different context can be created if the son-in-law answers the question, since he is less involved, less guilty, and less likely to reinforce the repetition unintentionally. By getting involved, he may also avoid a marital argument.

Information about the disorder and what to expect is an important part of the professional interaction. To provide the diagnosis without some education about the disorder is sufficiently unkind to the caregiver and other family members as to be unethical behavior. Families need some guidelines for what to expect and some assistance in comprehending where action is possible and where it is not. The provision of realistic hope is important as a guideline in this educational process. Unrealistic hope can push families into trying to assist older dementing persons to be what they used to be or to recover their memory and blame themselves for failure. An overly pessimistic view may lead to overlooking remaining strengths and to encouraging excessive dependency in the patient and excessive caretaking by the caregiver. For example, in early stages, some caregivers needlessly stay home in order to watch a dementing relative who does not yet need much watching.

Education should also involve some guidelines for what to expect next and what problems will be resolved with time. Suspiciousness and hostility from the patient, for example, are very disturbing for the family. Learning how to accept accusations without personalizing them and to understand them as a manifestation of memory loss rather than as a fundamental change in a previously loving relationship (e.g., a father accused his son of stealing the money because he forgot he spent it, not because he thinks the son is a thief) can be very helpful in extending a caregiving relationship through a time of crisis. It is also helpful for the family to know that this phase will pass as the disorder worsens. That is, eventually memory becomes so bad that the money is completely forgotten.

Referral to other resources is an important part of the assistance offered to caregivers of dementing persons. As I have elaborated elsewhere (1986a), mental health professionals tend to occupy a middle ground between medicine and social services. In the course of the dementing illness, the family will need assistance from all three systems, and the mental health professional must be able to provide accurate information about the local network of assistance and to assist in deciding how best to meet the family's needs with the available resources.

At various points, families will want to know about medical diagnostic clinics, ongoing medical care (some physicians withdraw after a dementing diagnosis is given), the various levels of twenty-four-hour care, respite services of all kinds (e.g., in-home care, day care, overnight care), public resources for health care and income supplements, transportation, casework, legal assistance for estate planning and guardianship, and more. Accuracy is highly important. One must not only understand the definitions of levels of care but the specifics that may make a particular residential care home, say, more accepting of a patient than most skilled nursing facilities would be. Planning for respite is often difficult in that families conceptualize their needs differently than the agencies that provide services. A family may want someone to watch over the demented relative for several hours, but someone's coming in and bathing the patient twice a week may be the service available.

Knowing what is available and affordable and knowing how to maximize the benefit of the service takes time and research. Given the complexity of the service network and the generally poor fit between what families want and what is available, simply passing out phone numbers amounts to maltreatment of the family member, who is likely to come full circle on the local "information and referral" circuit without getting needed services or finding someone who will candidly say that what he or she wants does not exist.

Psychotherapy for the caregiver can be an important part of the overall service plan and the needed support for the family system. In her study, Gray (1983) reported that the services most desired by caregivers were counseling and respite and that neither were available. There is growing evidence that primary caregivers are susceptible to depression and that depression is a causal factor in the decision to institutionalize (Poulschock and Deimling 1984). Brief, goal-oriented therapy that focuses on emotional release, realistic confrontation of the problem, decision-making, and stress management strategies can be of assistance to many caregivers. In many cases, one or more sessions with other family members may be very helpful in exploring and possibly resolving family issues and conflicts that may be complicating the problems of the principal caregiver. Some caregivers may need longer courses of therapy to resolve ineffective or counterproductive coping strategies (including persistent denial of the illness or using the patient's illness to avoid facing other personal and family problems) or to work through grief for the person and the relationship that has been lost even though the physical individual is still alive and present in the house.

The preceding discussion assumes that the situation was fairly uncomplicated prior to the dementing illness. But this is often not the case. Caregiver issues can become much more complex when the dementia is intruding into an already unhappy marriage. For example, after a number of therapy sessions, several caregivers have revealed that they had been considering divorce when the dementia was discovered and then felt obligated to stay and care for the dementing husband or wife. If the demented person was an abusive spouse or parent, this person's vulnerability and dependency will present complex problems for the caregiver who was a former victim. Some caregivers have had very dependent relationships in which they were used to depending upon the person they must now care for and make decisions for. Caregivers who have been passive and used to letting the spouse or parent make decisions may continue to do so long after the demented person no longer understands the questions, much less the decisions. Finally, some caregivers already have histories of depression, anxiety disorders, paranoia, and other psychoses. In all such more complex instances, the therapy will be more challenging and likely longer in duration. In fact, prolonged time spent in the very stressful caregiver role is likely to necessitate fairly lengthy intervention with the caregiver.

Case Example: Dealing with the Earlier Relationship

This conversation takes place well along in the therapy, after a rapport has been established and the client-caregiver (Dot) has been educated about dementia and has sometimes attended a support group. She has learned some strategies to alleviate the husband's anxieties when she is in another room of the house, but in spite of repeated attempts, she has not been able to schedule a regular afternoon of respite. The therapist knows that Dot has had one episode of depression early in the marriage, which was resolved without treatment over a two-year period. As the conversation begins, she is morose.

THERAPIST: Did you manage to take time off this week?
CLIENT: Of course not. [There is a pause. Therapist remains silent.] I just couldn't bring myself to leave the house.
THERAPIST: Why not?
CLIENT: I just don't think Amanda [a neighbor] can really take care of him.
THERAPIST: We've been over that ground several times. I don't think that's what's bothering you. [Client vaguely nods but keeps quiet.] I think you're afraid of something.
CLIENT: Afraid? What would I be afraid of? I need time off. I'd love it.
THERAPIST: Except you keep on not doing it. Look, what would happen if you really did take the afternoon off? Really think about it.

CLIENT: [after extended pause, eyes fill with tears while face looks afraid] I'd keep right on going.

THERAPIST: You're afraid you'd leave? But you've been taking care of him very well every day for six years. Why do you think you'd leave?

CLIENT: I was getting ready to when we got the diagnosis that he had Alzheimer's . . . then I had to stay.

THERAPIST: You don't blame yourself for the dementia?

CLIENT: No, it's just that I don't know when it started. Maybe it was never his fault that he was that way. I couldn't stand myself if I left him so helpless.

The conversation continues through this and many more sessions. It develops that her husband was verbally abusive constantly and physically abusive at times since the early years of their marriage. Her early depression was a reaction to an affair of his that ended when the woman married someone else. Dot had been passive and submissive most of the marriage but had decided to leave him after seeing her daughter's life improve after she divorced an abusive husband. Coincidentally, the daughter had encouraged the testing that determined the diagnosis of Alzheimer's disease. The mother feels unable to leave and now wonders how much of his earlier behavior was due to the early stages of the disease. This issue of history and probable relationship of various incidents to the disease is the topic of several sessions, as is the limits of her responsibility to her husband now. After deciding that she is not obligated to care for him because he had not cared well for her and that she could leave him and feel okay about it, she surprises the therapist by deciding to keep him at home. She does schedule two afternoons out a week and follows through on them.

The stress is not necessarily relieved by institutionalizing the patient since problems are going to continue after introduction to twenty-four-hour care. Also, the caregiver may have trouble coping with the mixture of relief and guilt that typically occurs with this move. He or she may become angry with the nursing home staff and will need assistance in understanding how much of this anger is real and justified and how much is displaced from intrapsychic concerns. Death of the patient is also likely to pose major problems of readjustment since death often comes after years of caregiving during which caring for the patient was the organizing principle of the caregiver's life.

Case Example: Coping with the Death of the Dementia Patient

After several years of connection with the team through support groups and occasional individual sessions, Alma comes for therapy after her husband rather unexpectedly dies.

ALMA: I feel so confused, I don't know what to think.
THERAPIST: How do you feel?
ALMA: You know, I miss him. Everyone seems to think I should be glad he's gone and I know he's better off. But I really miss him. [She begins to cry.]
THERAPIST: Of course you miss him; he was your husband; you loved him.
ALMA: [after crying a while] I knew you'd understand. You know, I do feel relieved, but mostly I miss him . . . not so much as he was this year, but I think of how he was before. I'm just not ready to do anything now.
THERAPIST: Do you need to do anything?
ALMA: I don't think so, but my friends and my daughter keep thinking up things for me to do.
THERAPIST: Friends and daughters often do that. But listen, you need time to grieve for him, and it's been so long since you had time for yourself, it'll take a while to remember what you enjoy doing anyway. Take the time.

This theme and considerable emotional expression continue for a few months, and then Alma returns to an active life at her own pace.

THERAPY WITH THE DEMENTED PERSON

In general, there is a strong assumption that psychotherapy is useless with demented individuals. They are assumed to be too cognitively impaired to benefit and, because of the nature of the disease, to decline cognitively regardless of therapeutic intervention. No doubt consideration of this topic is clouded by unscrupulous practices, such as that of mental health professionals who have consulted in nursing homes and billed for psychotherapy with individuals who are clearly incapable of speaking, comprehending what is said, or remembering from the beginning of the session to the middle much less from week to week. Clearly, for those dementing persons who are moderately to severely impaired, psychotherapy is of no value.

However, given the uncertainties of diagnosis in the early phases of dementia and most professionals' optimism with regard to diagnosing and treating depression, most people trained to work with the elderly are likely to engage in therapy with clients who turn out to be in early stages of dementing illnesses. Such experience calls attention to a number of characteristics of this population that are generally unremarked in the literature. In the early phases, memory may interfere with learning the therapist's name but not with recognition of the therapist and the development of the relationship. Emotional work is not much affected, but cognitive work, such as recalling behavioral assignments or interpretations, may require more time and more repetition than usual. Clients may arrive late or on the wrong day or have trouble getting to the session and then do quite well while in the session, even spontaneously referring to key points from previous meetings.

My experience has been that when there is no immediate threat of being institutionalized, people in the early phases of dementia often have an excellent sense of what is happening to their cognitive abilities. There is often much concern about the future, including the impact of the illness on themselves and on the family. Although there are notable exceptions, the general level of emotionality about the progressive disability is less than with heart patients or people who have progressive visual loss. In general, there is a group of people adjusting to significant disability and life change for whom therapeutic intervention may often be appropriate. As is true with, for example, cancer patients, psychotherapy is oriented to the emotional aspects of the patient's life and not to curing the disease. As research progresses and produces a laboratory test for Alzheimer's, the number of people who know that they will dement will increase significantly. One could predict that this new group who will know of the dementing process before the disease blunts emotional reactions may be much more emotionally distressed than current "early stage" patients tend to be.

Case Example: Therapy with a Demented Client

Herb is moderately demented and is seen in therapy sessions intended to help him cope with grief for his wife, who died about a year ago. His daughter has arranged for and pays for the sessions. This conversation occurs after about six sessions. He is familiar with the therapist but unsure of his function and does not recall his name.

THERAPIST: Did you get in any more trouble with your daughter about not eating?

HERB: No, we got that taken care of. I eat the meal on wheels right away and she calls to tell me about supper.

THERAPIST: What about at night? Do you have any more odd experiences at night?

HERB: [looking puzzled] No, I'm sleeping okay now.

THERAPIST: Well, let's talk about Clara now.

HERB: I keep wondering when she's going to get back. She's been gone a while now.

THERAPIST: Herb, Clara's dead. [Herb looks puzzled but seems to begin to remember.] You went to the funeral out at Maplewood. The ceremony was at Trinity Chapel.

HERB: [remembering and starting to cry] That's right, she's dead. A man should be able to remember his own wife is dead. [obviously feeling guilt] I did love her.

THERAPIST: I know you did, and you still do. It's not your fault it's hard to remember. You know you have trouble with that. Anyway, you do remember a lot about her. Tell me more about Clara.

The session continues with stories about Clara and crying off and on. The therapist has heard many of the stories several times. The sessions are continuing because Herb can be observed to show improved mood and, according to the daughter, improved self-care with each visit. Therapy is terminated after ten sessions. Herb remains in his home for four more years, with increasing support from the daughter, and then moves to a residential care home.

It is the therapist who is most likely to have difficulty in working with this dementing population. As is true with family caregivers, it appears to be more difficult to watch cognitive deterioration than to experience it. Since psychotherapists are, by selection and training, mentally oriented people, they are likely to find cognitive deterioration highly distressing. The knowledge that the person will continue to decline regardless of one's efforts will discourage many who cannot see the value of improving the lives of dementing persons for the next few years by an appropriately timed brief intervention. At the same time, there is the ethical necessity of constantly evaluating whether the person is still sufficiently intact to benefit, and deciding to terminate on this basis may produce a grief reaction in the therapist. Obviously, transference and economic issues can cloud this decision.

The question of when psychotherapy must end with the dementing patient is genuinely difficult. Goldfarb and Sheps (1954) report on effective brief interventions with a nursing home population who in retrospect sound to me to have been partly cognitively impaired. He describes brief contacts, directive interventions, and considerable reliance on transference to the therapist as father and as benevolent authority figure. For the therapist who can assess cognitive ability and enter into the world of the cognitively impaired, there may be substantial, as yet unexplored territory in simple, brief interventions that rely heavily on emotional impact and simple statements, with the therapeutic relationship itself reduced to a minimal level.

SELF-HELP GROUPS AND THE FAMILY OF THE DEMENTING INDIVIDUAL

Many of the ongoing needs of the caregiver and other members of the dementing family for information, emotional support, and specific suggestions for how to handle day-to-day problems can be met at least as well by self-help groups as professionals. Although often presented as an alternative to or substitute for professional caregiving (see Gartner and Riesman 1984), the self-help group might better be seen as a complement to professional help. Research suggests that the members of self-help groups have used and continue to use other sources of assistance (Knight et al. 1980) and that professionals value and often refer to self-help groups (Levy 1978). Self-help groups tend to emphasize support and positive interaction rather than interpretation and confrontation (Knight et al. 1980; Wollert, Levy, and Knight 1982). This low-key supportive style is just what is needed by many Alzheimer's caregivers.

In the Ventura Outreach Team, the need for such a service grew out of the realization that many caregivers of dementia patients were being seen in outpatient therapy and that much of our information and interventions were being communicated from one caregiver to another. In short, the therapists were often in the middle, functioning as purveyors of ideas and information. After educating ourselves about dementia, a workshop for families was planned and held on a weekend day to encourage attendance. There was a tremendously positive response and a request for ongoing support meetings. These meetings were led by various team members. The emphasis of meetings was on information, support, and sharing of ideas for coping with specific problems. The groups are not thought of as therapy groups, and individuals have been referred from therapy to the groups and from the groups to therapy as individual needs indicate.

The groups provide an environment for education about the disorder, recommendations for securing accurate diagnosis, referrals for needed resources, and mutually shared problem solving at the level described by Mace and Rabins's *36 Hour Day* (1981): "what do you do when . . . ?" There is also considerable opportunity for sharing and mutual emotional support. Group leaders can intervene to keep members from being judgmental or critical about interventions and to provide technically accurate information about the disorder and referral sources. The only negative reactions to the group have tended to come from the diversity of membership. Some persons whose relatives are mildly impaired can become upset at realizing how much more lies ahead. Others grow tired of going over what for them are past problems.

Fortuitously, our efforts began shortly after the initial organization of Alzheimer's Disease and Related Disorders Association (ADRDA) on the national level and the establishment of a chapter in nearby Santa Barbara County. Both the national group and the nearby chapter were helpful in our efforts to organize and supplied pamphlets, reading lists, and other types of information.

From the beginning, it was our hope that the group would become self-sustaining and develop its own leadership. For several years, this did not happen, and during this time, the Senior Outreach Team provided a telephone contact point, xeroxing, mailing lists and postage, and considerable consultation to the group. Although levels of support vary, discussions with other service providers at national conferences suggest that this experience is typical. While fulfilling the role of primary caregiver, the majority of people do not have the time or energy for organizational work. We also found that very few people want to stay with the group once the patient is placed outside the home or dies. The stress is sufficiently intense and of such long duration that many people want to move on to another phase of their lives when possible. The ones who do stay provide tremendous assistance to others by their work in ADRDA.

After several years of support by the outreach team, sufficient internal leadership developed to form a steering committee that included outreach team members in supportive rather than leadership roles. With advice and support from the neighboring chapter, the steering committee sought and obtained recognition from the national ADRDA as the Ventura County chapter in October 1985. With a president who had great organizational and fund-raising skills, the chapter was able to open an office on a part-time basis, take over the publicity for support groups and the distribution of informational materials, and sponsor several public education programs. Individuals on the outreach team continue to be involved as board members, advisory board members, and as support group leaders of some of the groups sponsored by the local chapter.

In short, the development of Ventura County ADRDA provides an example of mental health professionals recognizing a need for services that could be met by a self-help network, organizing that network, and providing substantial support to it over approximately four years until internal leadership developed that was able to turn it into a true, self-sustaining, self-help group. This program both served a community need and provided for optimally effective use of professional time.

CHANGES IN SERVICES FOR THE DEMENTED
IN THE 1980s

The outreach team must be constantly alert to changes in the community and in the service network that may alter the need for certain types of program responses by the team. A good program now will not necessarily be adequate five years from now.

For example, when the Ventura Outreach Team was starting its dementia program, Alzheimer's disease was relatively unknown, ADRDA had just begun, medical diagnosis was relatively poor, and it was common practice among medical, mental health, and social service professionals to ascribe most odd behavior among older persons to "senility," which was sometimes conceived of as a brain impairment and sometimes as a normal outcome of aging. In the intervening years, there has been a tremendous amount of attention given to Alzheimer's disease in both the national and regional media and a correspondingly increased awareness of cognitive impairment in the elderly as being due to disease. There has also been excellent continuing medical education in our area and in medical journals, with consequent improvement in diagnosis and good recognition of depression, malnutrition, medication interactions, and other acute causes of cognitive impairment in older people.

During the same period, however, there have been tremendous changes in the network of services for the elderly. Public services in general in California have been reduced with funding cuts at all levels. These cuts have tended to make publicly supported casework services and in-home supportive services of various kinds more scarce at a time when institutional services have been held constant in the face of a rapidly increasing aged population. Changes in Medicare policy during the same period have made in-home skilled nursing care more available for brief periods after acute hospitalization and have greatly increased the number of agencies offering assessment and referral services. Other changes in Medicare have encouraged acute medical hospitals to discharge patients earlier. In general, the result has been that a larger number of usually more physically frail older people are competing for scarcer resources, especially when they are no longer in need of skilled care as defined by Medicare regulations. For the demented, skilled care (in Medicare terms) is virtually never needed, and the net result of these changes is increased awareness, better diagnosis, and increased assessments but very little actual direct service available, especially to those of the lower middle class and below who cannot afford services or cannot afford private pay long enough to derive benefit.

In general, the Ventura Team has responded to this changing scene by reducing public education in this area, since it is widely available in the public communications media, and by down-playing our role in assessment of dementia, since diagnostic and assessment services are much more generally available. Instead, we have emphasized our role in providing support and counseling to the primary caregiver and in being available for consultation after the other services have come and gone. Since we do not need a referral immediately after hospital discharge, we often advise potential clients that we will make first contact a couple of months later when other support agencies can no longer be reimbursed for services. The needs in other parts of the nation are, of course, different, and each program must assess the quality and quantity of local services, the gaps in those services, and the local level of knowledge among the public and professionals concerning the dementing illnesses.

SUMMARY

This chapter has discussed a program for dementia victims and their families that was implemented in a community mental health center setting. The program included community education about dementing illnesses, assessment combined with education and referral, psychotherapy for family caregivers and in some instances psychotherapy with dementia victims who had mild to moderate cognitive impairment. Self-help groups, developed and supported by professional staff, became an increasingly important part of the service network. The self-help groups took over much of community education and used the outreach team for advice, assessment, and counselling services. As other programs and professionals have developed good assessment skills in diagnosing probable dementia, the team has concentrated more and more on psychotherapy and on assessment of difficult and mixed-diagnosis cases. While each team will need a unique profile of services to fit the needs of its own community, this model can provide a guide for ways that mental health services can assist dementia victims and their families.

In this chapter, and in others, I have often commented on the impact of working with these populations of the therapist as a major issue in adapting to work with the elderly. Chapter 7 explores this topic in more detail as a guide to planning the training and development of staff to work with the elderly, including the cognitively impaired elderly.

7

Effects on Therapists of Working with Older Clients

There is a general impression that working with older clients is difficult. But few authors have commented on specific difficulties, and there are very few reports from the field that describe the impact of working with older people on those who work with them. In describing reasons for avoidance of work with older clients, Kastenbaum (1964, 1978) has written eloquently of the impact of working with disability and dependency and with clients who are approaching death. In earlier work, I reiterated Kastenbaum's observations and suggested that these effects of work with the elderly may represent (at least for younger therapists) the result of confronting issues earlier than would occur in natural adult development (1986a, 1986b). I also described differences in countertransference issues for therapists working with older clients (1986a). These include the possibility of confronting unresolved parental issues, being inhibited by a positive grandparent countertransference, being fearful of death and illness, and avoiding sexual issues and recognition of erotic transference and countertransference.

In this chapter, I take a different, although not necessarily competing, view in describing my observations of the ups and downs of several therapists' reactions to work with older people. The reactions I describe here are generalized and based on the characteristics of the work as it has an impact on younger therapists. These observations are distilled from the reactions of a number of full-time and part-time mental health professionals who have worked with the elderly at Ventura County Senior Outreach, including clinical social workers, nurse therapists, psychologists, and psychiatrists. To a lesser degree, the responses of students in training (social work interns, psychology interns, and psychiatric residents) are used. There is no intentional implication that there is a developmental progression in the order in which these reactions are discussed.

EACH IS SO UNIQUE . . .

Many therapists without prior experience or training in working with elderly clients react positively to the work. They also generally comment with some surprise on how unique each older person is. Especially considering that virtually all of the therapists who have worked with Senior Outreach volunteered and were screened in the employment interview for a positive feeling about their previous experiences with the elderly, it is intriguing that they were surprised that the elderly have a variety of problems that can be dealt with in therapy.

This observation can only serve to underline how strong the expectation must be among mental health professionals that older people have essentially similar problems and that working with them cannot involve much variety. One suspects that among therapists who are less carefully selected the experience of therapy with older people may not overcome this prior expectancy and that some therapists may continue to perceive older people as essentially similar to one another.

WHAT DO I HAVE TO OFFER THEM?

Another common early reaction to work with older people is to question what the (especially younger) therapist has to offer to the older client. This reaction can come in at least two different forms. One is motivated by a perception of the clients as having more life experience and a wealth of knowledge and wisdom that are not yet available to the less mature therapist. This form of the reaction can be especially strong in therapists who are lacking in experience as workers, marriage partners, and parents as well as in overcoming adversities such as disability and chronic illnesses. In part, this expression of inadequacy may be mediated by the degree of emphasis that the therapist's theory of therapy and professional training places on the role of personal experience and the necessity of the therapist's being (in some sense) ahead of the client. Two possible resolutions of this dilemma include the therapist recognizing both the strengths and limits of the expertise he or she does have: that is, therapists presumably are expert in the work of psychotherapy, which, as a change process, depends not so much on the therapist's having personal experience of the content of the client's problem(s) but only on skill in managing the process. In this sense, I have at times told clients that I do not know the answer to their problems but that I am sure I will recognize their discovery of the answer.

Another potential solution is to see oneself as a conduit for information and possible solutions to problems gained in formal education in gerontology as well as in clinical experience with other older clients. In any case, helping other clinicians to overcome these barriers often amounts to assisting them in discovering their own competency as therapists with this population.

The other manifestation of the question "What do I have to offer them?" is a sense of being overwhelmed by the enormity and "realness" of the problems faced by older people. Many older people are coping with the reality of the deaths of loved ones and the approach of their own death and are adjusting to limited income, socially defined roles and options, and to significant functional limitations of physical disability and chronic illness. As was discussed in chapter 4, therapists are often ushered (unfortunately, often for the first time) into the world of hospitals, nursing homes, prosthetic devices, catheters, feeding tubes, funeral parlors, and so on. In this realm, any doubts that the therapist has about personal adequacy or about the efficacy of therapeutic listening, emotional expression, alternative interpretations, the problem-solving process, changing reinforcement schedules, or simply "being there" are likely to surface in powerful ways. With appropriate guidance and support, the new therapist can learn to value therapy as one source of help for people in dire circumstances and to recognize that therapy can be of major help in some instances, of moderate help in some, and of no help in others. In other words, like other sources of help, psychotherapy is neither a panacea nor a worthless pastime but is of value to those who need what it has to offer.

For example, it may take a special person to sit with an elderly man who is facing certain progressive visual loss and blindness and ask if he would like to talk about the depression he feels. It no doubt requires a special perspective to suggest that he may be able to exercise some control over how bad the rest of his life will be and to admit that the choices are bad and less bad. The process of working with older clients in facing death and illness does tend to alter and inform one's work with younger clients; it can expand one's concept of when hope is realistic and create a different sense of how long the lifespan is and so how much time there may be to develop and work out problems. As psychotherapy with older adults matures as a discipline, it may well come to influence the practice of therapy with younger adults.

In some instances, of course, the sense of therapeutic impotence in the presence of older clients may reflect a countertransference issue that will require more than education and experience to overcome. It may necessitate careful clinical supervision and possibly personal therapy for the clinician. While my own experience suggests that this is a relatively rare phenomenon, missing countertransference when it does occur has harmful consequences for clients and for the clinician. Countertransferential impotence tends to arise with clients who remind the therapist of his or her own powerful grandparent or older parent figures or in situations that evoke unresolved issues, such as the placement of a beloved grandparent in a nursing home or the death of a grandparent or parent from a specific disease.

ARE WE ALONE IN OUR CONCERN FOR THEM?

Mental health workers serving older adults can feel isolated in a variety of contexts. Younger therapists may be relatively isolated from other young adults, both in terms of work and social contacts and in terms of the worldview conditioned by work in the aging service sector. Within the latter context, the concern with mental health problems and the mental health approach to conceptualizing problems are relatively new, as are the disciplines involved. Geriatric psychiatrists, psychologists, and, in particular, those who believe that outpatient therapy is useful with the elderly are a rare phenomenon. Social workers and nurses are more common, but they usually function in casework and home nursing roles rather than as clinical social workers and mental health nurses. Some may feel a need to explain their presence, which in turn can raise questions for them about their work.

In short, the person who works in the field of mental health and aging may often lack a clear reference group to bolster his or her identity. When a program is new, staff are almost certain to be alone on the local level. The sense of isolation can accelerate dissatisfaction by leading staff to question the value of their work or the assumptions on which the work is based. That is, the more intensely aware one is of being isolated and of the scarcity of others doing similar work, the easier it is to wonder if the work is worth doing or if the assumptions about the success of psychotherapy with older people are accurate.

While the effects of this feeling can easily become pervasive and undermining if ignored, the solutions are straightforward. Opportunities must be created to interact with others who are in the same or similar types of work. This can be accomplished through staff's attending professional conferences, training sessions, and (if need be, creating) regional or statewide meetings on a regular basis with other outreach teams and persons in the mental health and aging field.

On a day-to-day basis, support within the team is quite important. Leadership can also actively foster a sense of pride and accomplishment in the team's pioneering a new service concept in a locality and keep alive a creative spirit in the outreach work.

WHY CAN'T I KEEP MY CLIENTS ALIVE?

Having worked to encourage a spirit of therapeutic optimism and to sell the community on the value of psychotherapy, it is easy to implicitly overvalue the effects of therapy with older people. Clinicians may feel that their work is inadequate when a person who has received a considerable investment of therapeutic effort dies, worsens in the course of a chronic illness, or requires more intense care. Although it is unlikely that any psychotherapist thinks that therapy can prevent death or reverse the course of a progressive illness, our hopes for clients are often positive in a nonspecific manner, and it is only when the disappointment is experienced that the unrealistic expectation is identified.

In the same way that the client must be guided to be neither overly pessimistic nor unrealistically optimistic in the face of these major challenges in life, the therapist must steer a course between therapeutic nihilism in work with older clients and an optimism that borders on grandiosity. Goals must be carefully constructed to be realistic or to err slightly in the optimistic direction but not to set up either client or therapist for failure. There is also an often subtle but critically important difference between stating that improving a client's emotional state in the last few weeks of life or that helping someone to come to terms with a chronic and progressive condition is a valuable goal for psychotherapy and *feeling* successful when that is the outcome and then learning of or witnessing the client's deterioration or demise. Within our society, there is sufficient belief in the importance of positive attitude in combatting illness and in prolonging life that it can be all too easy a step to expect that attitude change should result in healing. In some instances, there may be, in fact, dramatic changes in health status that were initiated by or mediated by changes produced in therapy. In other cases, the client's attitude improves, and the client dies happier.

The solution to this issue is clearly the maintenance of an appropriate and realistic attitude about the value of psychotherapy. Achieving and maintaining this attitude requires self-monitoring and monitoring by teammates. It also requires a willingness to engage in mutual clinical supervision and to process these complex and often painful issues with one's workmates. It is quite possible that personal therapy may be necessary at times in order for the therapist to adequately handle the feelings elicited by constant confrontation with these issues. One aspect of lack of training about aging among psychotherapists and the pervasiveness of age stereotypes is that those of us who have sought personal therapy have had difficulty in finding a therapist who did not view continuing to work with the elderly as a masochistic decision. Our therapists, of course, had decided to work with other practicing therapists, who are usually considered to be even easier and/or more rewarding than the typical private practice clientele.

DO SENIOR OUTREACH WORKERS AGE FASTER?

While unlikely to be true in the literal sense, experience suggests that long-term, full-time work with older clients may, in fact, produce a sense of psychological aging characterized by some of the following symptoms: concern with forgetfulness and anxiety about losing one's memory; atypical concern with prevention of chronic illness; atypical interest in retirement benefits and financial security after retirement; a precocious concern with the relative quality of various ways to die; an early interest in selecting and appointing surrogate decision-makers to handle one's estate and health care decisions; and an unnatural concern with and attention to one's own aging process.

All of these specific concerns point to a more general fact about working with the elderly: Such work, by its very nature, implies a confrontation with late-life issues earlier in life than is commonplace. In the typical course of development, most people seem relatively unaware of the aging process and the finiteness of life until they witness it in their parents' aging process or until personal physical limitations bring the point home. Since therapy involves forming intimate relationships with clients, the therapist does confront such issues in a rather personal way and in greater variety and with greater constancy than is true of most people. The majority of people see mainly their parents' example and then are affected perhaps only for as long as each crisis lasts; or they may be sufficiently practiced at denial to miss even the growth potential in acknowledging their own parents' aging.

Aside from the rarity of the experience, one could question whether younger adults—meaning anyone one ten to fifteen years or more behind the client—possess the personal resources to confront these questions with equanimity. Older people confront only their own aging and have the benefit of their prior experience with parents' aging and a lifetime that may have crystallized their concepts of themselves and thus given them a clear sense of their strengths in the face of adversity. They have experienced themselves in a variety of roles (worker, parent, friend, etc.) and are likely to have found themselves competent in many of these roles. They have had some experience with illness and burying relatives and friends; they have seen relationships of all kinds form, change, and end. In confronting the problems of old age earlier than is normative, the younger therapist may be confronting them without sufficient personal preparation. In so doing, the young therapist may be vulnerable in the same way that we think of others who confront events "too early" as being: for example, teenage mothers, young widows or widowers, young adults with considerable management responsibility, and others.

In confronting such issues "too early," the therapist risks becoming overwhelmed and falling into a depression or a sense of lost identity or lost adulthood or middle age. (The parallel here is to children who are forced to become adults early and so miss out on childhood.) One would suspect this is especially likely when training fails to provide sufficient personal as distinct from intellectual preparation or when the job provides insufficient personal support.

However, even when the therapist successfully copes with this challenge, it may come at the price of maturing early in a psychological sense and therefore becoming alienated to some degree from one's own contemporaries. In this sense, even the successful teenage mother is no longer a normal teenager; nor is the young widow a typical young woman. In a similar sense, the young therapist working with older people is incapable of the naive unawareness of the possibility of death or of chronically disabling physical illness in the way that others of his or her age may be. Just as the teenage mother may find boys her own age immature, the therapist with aging experience may find it difficult to take seriously the struggles for meaning and identity that can characterize younger adult clients.

The challenge for the developing profession is to articulate more clearly the processes that will enable therapists to meet late-life challenges early and to build in coping ability and support in training and work settings. At present, we appear to rely on those who choose the profession possibly with accidental preparation provided by their having had unusual contact with grandparents or older parents or atypically early experience with chronic illness and death.

WHEN HOME AND WORK COLLIDE

Much of the above speaks to the personal difficulty of coping with the challenges that face older people. This difficulty is most clear and coping failures become most common when the professional faces the same problems at home as at work. When parents become frail or begin to die, when an older spouse retires, when the workers' family is facing placement decisions, the separation between work and private life becomes virtually impossible to maintain, and coping is likely to break down for some period of time.

The response to these crises is as varied as the individuals experiencing them. From the program viewpoint, however, there needs to be greater than usual acceptance and support of the stressed worker and flexibility with time off and with assignment of workload. There must also be careful supervision to assist the worker in avoiding transmitting his or her own sense of helplessness to clients and overgeneralizing the lessons learned in the personal crisis to all clients facing similar crises.

SUMMARY

This overview of hazards of work with the elderly may present an unpleasant view of that work. It should be pointed out that there are rewards both extrinsic and intrinsic and that much of mental health work involves similar difficulties. (For instance, I do not know whether work with older people is more difficult or easier than work with adolescents, with substance abusers, with veterans etc.) It is important, however, that these hazards be considered in selecting and training people for this work and in planning services that maintain an effective core of people able to work with the problems of later life.

Part II

INTEGRATING RESEARCH AND PRACTICE

As I discussed briefly at the end of chapter 2, the Ventura Senior Outreach Team has been characterized and guided from the beginning by a strong interest in research and program evaluation. The remaining chapters of this book bring together previously published material from that research and evaluation effort as well as new data on our outreach to Hispanic elderly. Because research programs in community-based, service-oriented settings are somewhat rare, some comments on the way in which this one developed and the benefits for service provision are in order.

Having been trained as a clinical psychologist in a research-oriented department of psychology, I have been preoccupied since my days as a graduate student with the question: "How do we know what we think we know?" As I became acquainted first with the literature on practice in gerontology and later with the aging services network, this concern intensified. I have repeatedly found that much of what is believed in gerontology practice has very little documented basis in either research or clinical practice. For example, in my first review of the literature on psychotherapy with the elderly, I commented on the persistence of the question "Is therapy possible with the elderly?" This question was continually asked despite several decades of clinical reports of successful therapy with older clients.

Another example is reflected in the studies reported in the next chapter. The research on therapists' attitudes toward the elderly was begun in the full expectation that therapists would be biased against the elderly and that the results of our study would lead to training programs to change that bias. Instead, we found no evidence of bias among therapists in our mental health department or of a relationship between attitude toward the elderly and service delivery to older populations. For our purposes, this finding was enough to suggest a change in direction for our outreach efforts. Without this data, however, we might well have spent many hours over several years doing programs to change therapists' attitudes toward the elderly without benefit to our program or to the field more generally.

The same sort of practical utility for program evaluation can be seen in chapters 9 and 10, which discuss evidence of success of targeted outreach efforts to specific referral agencies and types of populations. In addition to showing the effectiveness of outreach methods, these findings were helpful in guiding decisions about where to concentrate our community education efforts in order to benefit our clinical concerns.

In a different manner, the more conceptually oriented research already described in chapter 1 helped us to clarify our goals as a program by clarifying the definitions of frail elderly and the system of institutional care. The thinking that this research stimulated helped to define our objectives for each case and the limitations we faced in reaching the objective of delaying institutionalization, given the competing ideas of others who play an active role in the decision.

In short, examining what the program is doing in a quantitative way and basing decisions on that information has been an integral part of the development of the Senior Outreach program. Thinking about the results, writing about what was done, and therefore discussing the program with other people in both service and academic settings have helped to clarify important practical problems, to keep us honest, and to encourage program development. Our published scrutiny of our work has, I believe, encouraged other programs to adopt a spirit of realistic optimism about work with the elderly, and it has encouraged some to use psychotherapy and home visits. The feedback from field applications has been useful to some in academic settings who are developing theoretical concepts about services to older adults.

One particular aspect of the feedback from the academic community has consistently intrigued me and has practical implication for program planning as well as writing. Operating in two disciplines, gerontology and psychology, has at times put me in the interesting situation of being told by one that a finding is too radical to report without more documentation while being told by the other that the finding is so widely known and accepted as to be unworthy of report. For example, gerontology reviewers often found the results of research on therapists' attitudes radical in view of the great number of articles asserting the existence of therapist bias. Psychology reviewers, in sharp contrast, found the results to be subsumed under the well-known lack of relationship between attitudes and behavior.

I cite this example not to carp about review practices but to illustrate an important practical area in which gerontology research and writing did not draw on well-known general information in related fields. In both research and practice, there seems to be a regrettable tendency to reinvent the wheel when we try to understand and to serve older adults. Given the relative lack of knowledge about the elderly, we need all the information we can get. Related resources concerning younger adults with similar problems can be of great assistance in developing theory, research, practice, and policy.

This same lack of information necessitates a good flow of communication among service providers and researchers and theorists. Part of this communication needs to include the well-considered practical research and theoretical writing-up of case examples and examples that can only come from applied settings.

As a closing note to this introduction to the research section, I would like to acknowledge that there is a change in style and purpose from the first section. Those readers who are not research oriented may find the methods and results sections somewhat obtuse. I have decided to include them and to stick fairly closely to the originally published articles to enable those who are more research-minded to evaluate the basis for the conclusions stated in these chapters.

8

Studying Barriers to Therapy for the Elderly

This first research report follows the development and revision of our ideas about barriers to therapy for older adults. The research was done in the early days of the program, and the results informed our approach to dealing with this issue from nearly the beginning of the program.

For over thirty years, scores of articles have been written describing the underutilization of outpatient mental health services by the elderly (Rechtschaffen 1959; Oberleder 1966; Knight 1978–1979), yet the problem remains. Moreover, it is well established that the aged who do interact with the mental health system tend to do so in times of crisis and receive assessment and inpatient services, not treatment-oriented outpatient services (Zinberg 1964; Brothwood 1971).

Why is this so? Reviews of the literature on psychotherapy with the community-resident elderly often cite the negative attitudes of therapists toward the elderly (Butler and Lewis 1977; Knight 1978–1979; Kastenbaum 1964), arguing that therapists are prejudiced against elderly clients and exclude them from outpatient therapy.

This hypothesis is widely accepted in the field of gerontology. There are curious aspects to it, however. First, aside from a few inconclusive survey studies, there are no empirical data supporting this hypothesis. Coe (1967) describes a survey that documents negative attitudes among professionals. Dye (1978) reports a survey with more positive findings, but the samples are limited in various ways, and it is not clear what score would represent the cut off between negative and positive attitude toward the aged. Second, although there is a large and rich literature on general population attitudes toward the elderly (e.g., McTavish 1971; Nardi 1973; Bennett and Eckman 1973), therapist bias studies do not allude to this literature, use similar scales, or make direct comparisons between therapists and other groups. This lack of comparison further clouds the assessment of therapist attitudes as a barrier to mental health services. Are therapists more negative than anyone else? This question remains unanswered. Third, there has been no well-documented, successful attempt to change attitudes toward the elderly, especially among therapists. The focus on therapists' attitudes has

yielded the assumption that education will correct their (presumably) negative attitudes, but McTavish (1971) showed that training effects are equiv-
ocable, and another study showed a negative shift with training (Cichetti et
al. 1973). Finally, no studies directly assess the correlation between therapists' attitudes and the amount of services they offer to the elderly.

In sum, both the negativity of therapists' attitudes and their correlation
with service to the elderly are assumed, not demonstrated empirically.
There are studies that demonstrate that therapists' attitudes influence their
judgments about diagnosis and prognosis (Settin 1982); such studies, however, do not address the issue of barriers to therapy but of quality of
therapy.

This section describes a program of research that was designed to fill in
several of these gaps. Working within the framework of seeking to elimi-
nate barriers to therapy for the aged, the investigation began with a laboratory study using college students to check the properties of two scales of
attitude measurement. This study provides important information on the
similarities and differences between two ways of measuring attitudes and
provides a typically used sample to which therapists can be compared.
Experiment 2 replicated the reliability of these attitudes scales in a therapist population, compared attitudes of therapists to college students, and
tested the correlation of therapist attitude and utilization of therapy by the
aged. Experiment 3 built on the results of this second study and explored
barriers to outpatient services at a more systems-oriented level.

The investigator decided to use common measures of attitudes to maximize the comparability to other studies in the literature. Two types of
measures very commonly used to study attitudes in the general population
are Likert ratings of beliefs about the aged and various semantic differentials. The most commonly used Likert-type measure is Kogan's Older
Person (OP) Scale (Kogan 1961). The Silverman (1966) revision of the OP
Scale was used since it was demonstrated to have good predictive validity
in addition to the homogeneity and alternate forms reliability demonstrated
by Kogan. The evaluative portion of the semantic differential (SD) used by
Eisdorfer and Altrocchi (1961) was selected because of the evidence that
the measure is consistent across participant groups and concepts rated.
The rated target was defined as "old people in general" to maximize
similarity to the OP Scale.

These scales were correlated with a measure based on Tversky and
Kahneman's (1973) availability heuristic. Their theory argues that judgments about groups are based on samples available in memory. Since
availability in memory may be influenced by recency, dramatic nature of
examples, and semantic associativity, attitudinal judgments about elderly
would be based on whether a particular participant recalled frail, demented

elders or dramatic examples of successful elders when the judgement is required. Recalled persons could be public figures or personal acquaintances. After recall, the participants were asked to rate each remembered person for ease of recall and to rate each person "by indicating the extent to which you would like to age the way this person has aged." This rating of the memory sample was used to assess the positive evaluation of the recalled persons. This memory sample is used here as a test of types of elders available in memory and so of personal experience with the elderly.

EXPERIMENT 1: MEASURING ATTITUDES TOWARD THE ELDERLY AMONG YOUNG ADULTS

Method

Participants. Thirty-six undergraduates in a class on abnormal psychology at a midwestern university were participants in this study. Four turned in incomplete data and were excluded from analysis. Twenty of the respondents were female, mean age was 21.1 years, and most (28) were junior- and senior-level college students. Hometown size was split between under 50,000 (14) and over 50,000 (18) groups.

Materials. The Kogan OP Scale is scored so that a high score reflects a positive attitude. Scores could range from 16 to 80. In the semantic differential, six adjective pairs were repeated in reverse order so that interitem reliability could be measured. All SD scores were based on the nonredundant items. A higher score reflects a more positive attitude. Scores could range from 13 to 65.

Students were asked to recall ten elderly, as I have described above. For each old person recalled, the respondents were asked to write down initials, relationship to respondent, and best guess of the older person's age. The mean rating of this sample and the percentage of the sample rated over the neutral rating (5 or higher) on the 7-point scale constituted two more measures in this study. Demographic variables such as sex, age, size of hometown, and level of education were requested in a brief questionnaire.

Results

Cronbach's α was used to assess the internal consistency of the two attitude scales. For the OP Scale α (16) = .80 and for the SD Scale

α (13) = .85. The average interitem correlation (using Fishers z transformation) of the six repeated items in the SC Scale was .83.

The two scales were highly intercorrelated—r = .60, ($p.$ < .001)—supporting the concept that both are measures of the underlying construct of attitude toward the elderly. Several interesting differences between scales were, however, discovered. No significant differences in attitudes were found in comparisons for sex, race, class standing in college, participant age, or small versus large hometown. (There was a statistical trend, $F(1,30)$ = 4.02, p < .06, with smaller hometowns yielding more positive ratings than larger ones on the OP Scale.) Out of fourteen tests of relationships to demographic variables, there was one significant finding: the SD Scale (but not the OP) was significantly correlated with number of living grandparents: r = .40, p < .01.

Since the attitude scales are correlated, the partial correlation was computed between each attitude scale and the evaluation of the memory sample, holding the other scale's variation constant. For the SD Scale, the partial correlation was r = .56, p < .001, for the OP Scale r = −.16, N.S.

Discussion

These findings demonstrate that these measures of attitude toward the aged have a high degree of internal consistency in this population. Their significant interrelationship argues for these two quite structurally different scales tapping the same construct of attitude toward the aged. As one would expect in such differently constructed scales, there is also considerable divergence between them, with measures being responsive to differing aspects of the expression of attitudes toward the aged.

The fact that the SD Scale (a more evaluative/affective measure in structure) correlates with the number of living grandparents and with the evaluation of elders available in memory suggests that this scale is more related to personal experience with the aged. Two other studies using semantic differentials and experience with the aged support this finding (Rosecranz and McNevin 1969; Bekker and Taylor 1966).

The OP Scale, directed toward the belief component of attitudes, is less directly affected by personal experience. These results call attention to the possibility that these scales measure differing aspects of the dual components of attitude (belief and evaluation). Thus, these results support both the concept that there is an underlying common dimension of "attitude toward the aged" and that this construct is sufficiently complex and the measures sufficiently dissimilar to be affected differently.

EXPERIMENT 2: ATTITUDES OF PSYCHOTHERAPISTS
TOWARD THE ELDERLY

Method

Participants. The sample of therapists included 66 mental health workers—psychiatrists ($N = 7$), psychologists ($N = 6$), clinical social workers ($N = 14$), psychiatric nursing staff ($N = 7$), rehabilitation therapists ($N = 7$), and psychiatric technicians ($N = 10$)—in a community mental health center in Southern California. Male therapists were 28 in number, and the mean age of the sample was 40.4 ($s.d. = 9.86$).

Materials. The attitude measures were the ones used in Experiment 1. In addition to information such as job class and work site, participants were asked to report total clients seen in the last month and clients aged 60 and over seen in the last month, to indicate desire for change in extent of clinical contact with the aged on a 5-point scale, and to rate their interest in working with aged clients on a 5-point scale.

Results

The interitem homogeneity (measured by Cronbach's α) of these scales in the therapist population was α (16) = .72 for the OP Scale and α (13) = .85 for the SD Scale. The interitem correlation for the six repeated SD items was .69. These internal consistency measures were high and comparable to those found with college students in Experiment 1. The correlation between Kogan's OP and the SD Scales was moderate but significantly different from zero, $r = .27$, $p < .05$. The direct test of difference between this correlation and the corresponding one in Experiment 1 yielded a non-significant difference, $z = 1.86$, N.S.

The direct comparison of therapists' and college students' attitudes toward the aged showed no significant difference on the SD Scale and a significant difference on the OP Scale, which indicated that therapists have the more positive attitude ($t(96) = 3.01$, $p < .01$).

Correlations were computed for each attitude scale with percentage of clients seen in the past month who were over 60, desire for change in clinical contact with the aged, and self-rated interest in working with the aged. For these correlational calculations, fifteen therapists assigned to children's programs were excluded from the sample since their contact with the aged of necessity was zero. The six correlations ranged from $-.17$ to $+.19$, and none was significantly different from zero.

Relationships between amount of clinical contact with the aged and other variables were also tested. The correlation of therapist age and contact with the aged ($r = -.11$) was not significant; nor were there significant differences between male and female therapists or among disciplines on clinical contact with the aged. The sole significant finding was that work site (which outpatient clinic the therapist worked in) was a significant determinant (F [4,46] = 3.80, $p < .05$), accounting for 25% of the variance in clinical contact with the aged.

Discussion

The replication of the reliability and interrelatedness of the two measures of attitudes is an important step in understanding attitudes per se. The finding of similar degree of correlation between the scales, as in Experiment 1, suggests that there is divergence between these scales with therapists, as there was in the college student sample (probably due to the different structures). The scales were as reliable in the therapist sample as in the college student sample, and this finding can open the door to more direct comparisons of these groups using the same attitudinal measures.

The direct comparison of groups' attitudes toward the aged yields the finding that therapists' beliefs about the aged (reflected in the OP Scale) are more positive than those of college students, while the component of attitude that is more evaluative and more related to personal experience is not different from that of college students. These observed differences could be because (1) therapists have a more positive set of beliefs about the aged than does the general population; (2) therapists gain a positive change in beliefs (but not the evaluative component of attitudes) with training, since in the past this community mental health center had been the site of training sessions sponsored by the Andrus Gerontology Center; or (3) measured sample characteristics were not related to attitudes toward the aged. The most provocative finding of this experiment is a negative result; namely, the lack of significant correlation among attitude measures and degree of clinical contact with the aged, reported desire for change in clinical contact, and interest in working with the aged. Two conclusions that cannot be differentiated by these data are possible:

1. These attitude measures are reliable but not valid measures of attitude toward the elderly (they possess internal consistency but do not

correlate with other variables, such as working with the elderly, with which attitudes ought to correlate); or,

2. These scales are good measures of attitudes, but attitudes are not important correlates of clinical work with the aged.

Within the context of literature on psychotherapy with the aged, it is radical to argue that therapists' attitudes may not be an important factor in the degree of clinical work with the aged. More than thirty years of literature has assumed both the negativity of therapists' attitudes and that these negative attitudes are a major barrier to the aged obtaining access to mental health services. Dozens of educational programs have attitude change as a principal goal. The results of this study, however, show that the assumption of relationship between therapist prejudice and therapy accessibility is just an assumption, and an incorrect one at that.

If not attitudes, then what are the barriers to therapy for the aged? Experiment 2 suggests that work site is a major determinant of contact with the aged. In fact, it accounts for 25% of the variation in clinical contact with the aged. This is a robust finding in the social sciences. In this study, the five work sites are different in terms of a variety of features, including location in community, physical features of the clinic, administrative commitment to problems of the aged (some clinic directors were active in department-wide community service programs for the elderly, others were more identified with children's services, services to psychotic young adults, etc.), accessibility to public transportation, handicap access, proportion of elderly in the local catchment area, and many other features. Given the large number of differences and the small number of sites, it is not possible with the data from this study to clarify what about some of the sites leads to greater service to elders. It can be recommended, however, that future research would do well to focus on this question rather than on therapist attitudes. A national survey of clinical psychologists by Settin (1982) provides independent support for the importance of work site as influencing work with the elderly.

This finding that work site is an important determinant of work with the aged invites the application of a model that allows for examination of the "barriers to therapy" problem at a more macrolevel than the inside of the therapy room. Intervention might then change from educational programs that attempt to change attitudes of individual therapists to system-level interventions that change physical environment, agency policy, staff-client interaction, and the social climate.

EXPERIMENT 3: MANAGEMENT VARIABLES AS
PREDICTORS OF OUTPATIENT USE BY ELDERLY

As we have seen in the previous two experiments, the barriers to mental health service utilization by older people would seem to lie beyond the individual therapist. The finding that work site accounts for a large part of the variance turned our attention to system-level variables and to factors identified by community mental health as important to service utilization by other underserved groups.

The community mental health movement has long been concerned about delivering mental health services to underserved populations. Reasons for underservice have been analyzed in terms of lack of availability of service, lack of awareness of services, lack of acceptability of services to the client population, and lack of accessibility (Little 1976). Gatz et al. (1980) have emphasized the interacting roles of client variables, therapist variables, and system variables in understanding the barriers to therapy for the aged. These analyses are complementary in that awareness and acceptability are client variables.

Among these three domains, there is reason to select system variables for specific consideration. Client variables are being shown to be less important than previously throught, probably due to cohort effects, and relatively easy to overcome (Gatz et al. 1980; Garfield 1978). The previously reported experiments in this chapter weaken the argument for the importance of therapist variables. This leaves system variables as a likely candidate to explain the underservice to the elderly, and, as noted by Gatz et al. (1980), the mental health services system for the aged has many inadequacies.

Within the analysis proposed by Little (1976), availability of services takes a role logically prior to other variables; simply stated, if the service is not available, then it matters little whether it is acceptable and it can hardly be accessible. The current state of services to the elderly strongly suggests that availability of services (whether or not services for elderly are offered) may well be a major factor in the underservice of elderly by mental health systems.

The focus of the third study is the administrative policy variables that reflect the decision to offer services to the elderly through a community mental health center. Every center maintains some level of a management information system that contains information on type of clients served, population characteristics of the catchment area, activities and deployment of agency staff, fiscal information, and agency priorities (Little 1976; Broskowski 1976). By examining these management variables, it becomes possible to ask such questions as: How many staff are assigned to work with elderly? What priority do services to elderly have in agency planning? Are services offered through special age-specific programs or in regular centers? Do staff have specialized training? Each of these questions measures a different aspect of the administrative decision to offer services and the method by which services are offered. These management variables can then be correlated with proportion of elderly using inpatient versus outpatient care to determine which management strategies are strongly related to service utilization in those two modalities.

The selection of specific management variables was based on an analysis of the management issues likely to impact on availability of services to the aged and a consideration of what information is readily available in the management information systems of mental health programs in California. (Note that California has more than two million older citizens, or 9.4% of all older Americans, the largest population in any one state according to the 1980 Census.) The questions asked in this study are basic to making services available to the elderly:

1. Are staff assigned to work with the elderly? How many?

2. Are these services offered through a specialized program or in generic programs (i.e., as part of regular adult outpatient services)?

3. What types of services are emphasized (e.g., screening, psychotherapy, medication)?

4. Do staff have specific training in aging? At what level?

5. What rank do geriatric staff hold in the agency?

6. What proportion of inservice training, community education, and consultation time is devoted to age-related work?

7. How many elderly citizens serve on the mental health advisory board?

8. In planning, what is the ranked priority of services to the elderly?

This study investigated the relationship of each of these management variables to inpatient and outpatient utilization of mental health services by elders in the State of California.

Method

Participants. The units of analysis for this study are the fifty-eight Short-Doyle programs in the State of California. (Short-Doyle is the enabling legislation for the state-funded, locally controlled system of community mental health centers in California.) Survey questionnaires were directed to the executive directors of these centers. There is considerable variation in size of counties (from rural to major metropolitan areas) and in size of mental health departments. Every department in the state of California was included.

Measures. The survey questionnaire included the management questions listed above, all of which provide information that is requested in the annual plans prepared by each program for the State Department of Mental Health. The questionnaire also requested the number of clients served by age (0 to 18, 19 to 64, over 65). In addition, the proportion of the county population over 65 was requested since it was expected that this variable would be an important moderator-predictor of service utilization (that the counties with high percent of elderly would have higher utilization).

Procedure. The questionnaires were mailed to all fifty-eight executive directors of Short-Doyle programs with a cover letter explaining that the study's purpose was to determine reasons for variation in utilization of therapeutic services by the aged and promising confidentiality of individual program results and a summary of the findings. After eight weeks, a second letter was sent with a second copy of the questionnaire to those who had not responded. This procedure yielded a 69% return rate ($N = 40$).

Results

Since both children's services and services to the aged are often conceptionalized as special services to special populations, there is room for competition between these programs, which could result, for example, in departments with good children's programs showing a low percentage of elderly in total client load. For this reason, utilization rates by aged (over 65) were calculated both as percent of total client load and percent of adult caseload. These measures were essentially identical ($r = .99$), and so, percent of adult caseload was used in subsequent analyses.

An obvious potential factor that would be expected to correlate with utilization of mental health services by the elderly is percentage representation of elderly in the county's population. However, this did not turn out to be true. For outpatient utilization, the correlation between county population over 65 and client load over 65 was $r = .096$, N.S., and for inpatient service, $r = .007$, N.S. Thus, the utilization of mental health services by the aged is statistically independent of their proportional representation in the general population. The correlation of inpatient and outpatient utilization rates was also not different from zero, $r = -.051$, N.S.

Tests were performed on the eight variables previously listed for their influence on utilization of outpatient services and on utilization of inpatient services. Since sixteen significance tests were performed, the type one error for each test was set at .01 to minimize the likelihood of reported results being due to chance. Two variables were significant. The number of staff assigned to geriatric services was a significant predictor of outpatient utilization, $r = .575$, $p < .0001$, but was not related to inpatient utilization. The variable thus explains 33% of the variation in outpatient utilization across the counties. The percentage of advisory board members over 65 was a significant and an inverse predictor of inpatient utilization, $r = -.393$, $p < .01$, but unrelated to outpatient utilization. This explains 15% of the variance in inpatient utilization.

Discussion

Two negative findings have potentially important implications for understanding the findings of this investigation and for thinking about the underservice of the elderly more generally:

1. Inpatient utilization is statistically independent of outpatient utilization; and

2. Both measures of service use are independent of proportion of elderly in the county's population.

The former finding fails to support the argument that increased outpatient services would lead to decreased inpatient usage. In order to decrease inappropriate use of inpatient mental health services, services will need to be designed for that population presently using those services. This is not to argue that outpatient services are not necessary services for the elderly but that they should not be provided with the expectation of substituting for inpatient programs. As an alternative, one might expect programs intentionally designed to substitute for inpatient services to reduce inpatient use. For example, Penner et al. (1983), describe a behavior skills-training program in a day treatment center that successfully returned state hospital patients to the community.

The finding that services to the elderly are uncorrelated with the proportion of elders in the county population strengthens the argument that it is management strategies (or some attribute of the mental health services) that makes the difference in delivery of service to the elderly and not simply the prevalence of elders in the population or other such "market

122   *Integrating Research and Practice*

indicators." That is, simply having large numbers of seniors in the catchment does not lead to high utilization.

The predictor of outpatient services utilization discovered in this investigation was the number of staff assigned to work with the elderly. This suggests that a key factor in increasing service delivery to the elderly is to assign staff to deliver such services. Given a basic sense of professional responsibility and knowledge of basic community mental health outreach methods, this has apparently been enough to increase service use by this underserved group. The converse interpretation of this correlation (that increased demand by elderly leads to assignment of specific staff to work with them) is weakened by three observations:

1. Since service use is not predicted by proportion of elderly in the catchment, and since elderly have generally underused services, it is difficult to explain this demand for staff at some centers;

2. Even if this unexplained increased in demand did occur, there is no obvious reason for management to react by assigning specific staff to deliver services—it seems more likely that services would be delivered by generic outpatient clinic staff (a sudden increase in the use of services by, say, wives of Vietnam veterans would not create a special staff assignment or even be likely to be noticed); and

3. The case histories of three such programs clearly demonstrate that the sequence was recognition of low rates of services to aged, the decision to implement a program, and then higher rates of service after specific staff assignment (Ruffin and Urquhart 1980; Selan and Gold 1980; Knight, Reinhart, and Field 1982).

A closely related issue, the specialized training of staff in gerontology, could not be addressed since only seven programs had specifically trained staff.

The relationship of mental health advisory board representation and lower inpatient utilization is more subtle. Two possible explanations are:

1. Such representatives may serve to keep administrators alert to the potential high functioning of elders and so mitigate against a ready acceptance of inpatient assessment, medication, and placement of elders as the only appropriate service strategy; and/or

2. The presence of seniors on the advisory board of mental health may indicate an actively involved group of vocal senior advocates in the total community who have influenced that community to provide a richer social service and inhome support network for frail elderly, and this in turn might prevent their being admitted as patients.

These explanations are, of course, only suggested hypotheses, but they are testable hypotheses.

In conclusion, this exploration of the role of management variables as predictors of the use of mental health services by the elderly in California has uncovered two predictors that are quite strong (as measured by percent of variance explained) for the social services. These early results are encouraging with regard to the potential success of analyses focusing on system variables in resolving the problem of underservice to the aged by mental health centers. Research, policy analysis, and interventions at the systems level may well prove more fruitful than the previous focus on therapist and client variables.

SUMMARY

To recapitulate the major findings of the three studies reported in this chapter, the emphasis on therapist bias in the literature on barriers to therapy for the elderly would appear to be misplaced. The results reported here suggest that therapists may be, if anything, less biased against the elderly than college students are and that their actual delivery of service to the elderly is not determined by attitudes anyway. Preliminary results suggest that the actual barriers are more in system-level or management variables and include at least the decision to allocate staff to provide services to the elderly.

There may well be other important systems-level variables that influence service delivery to the elderly. The specific role of offering home visits in improving accessibility of services to the elderly is not addressed by these studies. The need for clinics that are both physically and socially acceptable to older clients has not been researched. The nature of factors that determine inpatient utilization have not been studied and so cannot guide programs that wish to have a real impact on reducing the use of psychiatric hospitals by older patients.

Finally, getting older people into the system of outpatient mental health care, or keeping them out of inpatient care, should not be the endpoint of programming or research. What happens to them after they connect with services is also important. Utilization issues should not be disconnected from process and outcome studies. The next chapter considers both the effectiveness of the Senior Outreach Team in increasing service use and the outcome of their therapeutic efforts in improving clients' mood and behavior and in preventing unnecessary institutional care.

9

Assessing the Mobile Geriatric Outreach Team

This chapter describes the evaluation of the achievement of the Senior Outreach Program at Ventura County Mental Health in terms of the program's twin goals of (1) making mental health services more accessible to the aged and (2) the prevention of inappropriate institutionalization. In addition, preliminary information on client improvement in therapy is reported.

Evaluation data on geriatric mental health programs are skimpy. Kahn (1977) has noted that evaluations of such programs often report treatment as outcome (i.e., case managers reroute patients from state hospitals to nursing homes and report fewer elderly in state hospitals). Frankfather (1977) described one mobile team that functioned largely to medicate nursing home patients who were acting out. Others (e.g., Blenkner, Bloom, and Nielson 1971) have questioned the efficacy of case-management-only models given the pervasive influence of custodialism and the desire to "protect" the frail elderly. In short, the simple existence of such a team does little to ensure more service, better service, or greater independence for the client group.

The Ventura model is different in a number of ways. The formation of the direct services team was preceded by a period of community education and staff training. The team thus began with both an aging network prepared for the team's advent and a mental health staff prepared for the work. This developmental history was described in more detail in chapter 2. In its organization, the program was an outpatient clinic within a community services department. This arrangement made possible a broad range of traditional and nontraditional mental health services. The staffing of the team was unusual in two ways: (1) The program manager is a clinical/community geropsychologist, and the director of community services was a community-oriented psychologist; (2) all staff were licensed professionals with previous experience in and commitment to community mental health. Staff included a clinical social worker, two mental health nurses, and a half-time psychiatrist in addition to the program manager. Finally, as an outpatient clinic with a specific goal of increasing the accessibility of services to the aged, the team is explicitly oriented to providing mental health outpatient treatment to the elderly on a fee-for-services basis. In other words, the program provides active treatment for clients and produces income for its department. In the beginning, it was expected that the second goal of prevention of institutionalization would be accomplished along with this first goal of making services accessible. The notion was that early detection, assessment, and treatment would prevent unnecessary institutionalization.

The services provided by the outreach team fall into three broad categories. First, provided on a community client-contact basis (a category that allows one or two visits at no charge and without diagnosis of mental disorder), assessment and referrals are offered to elders in crisis. This generally consists of a home visit by two team members of different disciplines who evaluate the client's problems and strengths and assist the client in seeking appropriate services from the local social service network. In the course of these visits, the team decides whether to begin outpatient therapy and/or medication visits. Brief therapy is the second broad component of the program. It has usually focused on depression, adjustment disorders, anxiety disorders, and paranoia. The third category is services to the aging network. These consist of consultation to various agencies, inservice training, community education, and assistance in program development.

Barriers to therapy described in the preceding chapter were specifically attacked. Part of the screening process for team members was an assessment of their positive feeling for the elderly. It was also made clear that the program was oriented toward maintaining maximal independence of the elderly client.

Lack of training was addressed by encouraging staff to read relevant literature on aging and mental health and to attend quality training sessions in the field. Field trips to other aging service programs were undertaken two or three times per year. All staff spent some of their early weeks on the job visiting local aging service agencies and getting acquainted with programs and staff. The inhibition of skills in geriatric cases was an issue frequently addressed in inservice training for other therapists. With respect to selection and training issues, I believe that it is easier to train open-minded licensed mental health personnel to work with the aged than it is to turn paraprofessional community workers into psychotherapists.

Client misconceptions about outpatient services were addressed during the early assessment visits. Clients were educated about the nature of therapy using the Orne and Wender (1968) anticipatory socialization for therapy model. Referral sources who were uncertain about referring to mental health were trained to use the anticipatory socialization outline as

a model referral strategy. Finally, I have developed a videotape presentation based on this model for use in community education and with clients
(1981).

The slowness of many elderly in identifying problems as psychological
has also been approached in an educational manner. Community education
programs are presented in various senior communities. These programs
start with more health-oriented concerns (sleeping problems, stress factors
in disease) and move gradually into psychological issues (depression, anxiety, memory loss). At the same time, the groups move from lecture style
to discussion style. After four years of preparing potential clients for therapy and presenting community education programs, it seems to me that in
most cases it is the aging-network provider rather than the older person
who is more reluctant to discuss mental health issues.

Environmental factors are also addressed by the team's structure and
procedures. The existing sliding-scale fee system for mental health services has proved adequate for client needs. Many clients pay nothing out of
pocket, others pay between $24 and $100 per year of service. No client
has turned us down due to inability to pay. Higher income clients are
generally referred to the private sector. Attempts to change public and
private insurance regulations are beyond our program's scope of control
and are not dealt with.

The problem of physical inaccessibility due to disability or lack of adequate mass transit is resolved by the use of home visits. Virtually all initial
visits are in the home, a practice common to most such teams. A more
unusual feature is that slightly over half of ongoing therapy visits also take
place in the client's home. The team considers this an essential part of the
program, and all team members (including the program manager and the
psychiatrist) make home visits. Our relatively young staff are healthy and
able to drive. Many of our clients are not.

Psychosocial accessibility is enhanced by the team's consultation and
education activities. Each team member provides training as well as case
and program consultation to aging-network agencies and cultivates referral
sources. The team also provides consultation and community education to
various advocacy organizations. By means of community education programs, discussion groups at congregate housing and meal sites, and personal availability, staff have become well known in the aging community as
a whole. This has generally been a two-step process in which the activities
described here make staff known to the relatively well elderly who inhabit
senior recreation centers, apartment houses, and meal sites. These elderly, in turn, become comfortable in referring more isolated elderly to us
when they can identify a staff member by name and with a personal
description (as opposed to saying "You need a psychologist"). Using the

same staff for clinical and community education activities, with the consequent direct generation of referrals, makes these activities cost-effective.

PROGRAM EVALUATION DATA

Since the beginning of the program, the client population has been largely female (68%), about one-third has been married, another third widowed, with the remainder divorced, separated, or single. Most clients (65%) are over 70 years old; a substantial number are over 80 (25%). Between March 1980 and February 1982, the program served an unduplicated count of 607 elderly. About 35% of these received outpatient therapy. The average number of therapy visits was 8.6.

The progression of outreach into the community of elders can be tracked in several ways. From the inception of the program, the percentage of clients over 80 steadily increased from 10.9% in the last six months of 1980 to 26.9% for the first six months of 1983. These figures serve as one rough indicator of the progress of the program in reaching the older and often more frail elderly.

The data on referral sources show two changes that are important indicators of improved program outreach. From the first year to the second year of the program, the proportion of referrals from acute care hospitals increased from 11% to 17.2%, indicating a measure of increased contact with the ill and disabled elderly. The percentage of referrals from senior service agencies also increased from 7% to 12.7%, indicating integration into the aging network. These changes also reflect an important aspect of program management. Information on referral sources is compiled regularly and compared to our concept of how the team should operate. These areas were targeted for increased consultation and education efforts at the end of the first year, and our efforts paid off in increased referrals from these sources.

One year after the program began, the team moved out of the mental health department's central offices and into offices in a heavily senior-populated area. In this location, our primary identification is as Senior Outreach Services, although our connection to mental health is neither denied nor concealed. The number of new contacts per month rose sharply at this time. Before the move, the average number of contacts was 21 per month. After the move, it was 32 per month, a statistically significant increase—$t(9) = 10.22, p < .001$.

General Evaluation

Client satisfaction with the program was assessed in June 1981 as part of the regular client satisfaction survey performed by the department's program evaluation office (Essex 1981). The comparison of senior outreach clients ($n = 15$) and outpatient service clients ($n = 217$) in a series of chi-square analyses shows that there are no significant differences in clients' satisfaction ratings between the two types of programs. Elderly clients in the outreach service and adult clients in the outpatient clinics are equally satisfied with the services they received.

Another measure of clients' reluctance to receive therapy is their "no show" rate. A time sampling of no-show rates at department clinics conducted in early 1982 (Essex 1982) demonstrated that senior outreach had the lowest no show rate in the department, with 1.2% for all no shows and 0.0% on intakes. (People can and do fail to keep home visit appointments by not being home or not answering the door.) The other outpatient clinics ranged from 5.7% to 12.9% for all no shows and from 9.5% to 32.2% on intakes. On this measure, elderly clients are more cooperative than are younger adults.

Therapists' ratings of clients' progress are another important source of information about the program's success. All clients in Ventura County Mental Health are rated at admission and again at discharge on the Global Assessment Scale, a measure of general mental functioning with specific behavioral descriptions of each ten-unit level (Spitzer, Gibbon, and Endicott 1976). For program reporting purposes, change in rating within a block (e.g., 70–79) is counted as no change, a change to a higher ten-unit block is improvement, and lower rating is negative change. Two clients who died were considered negative change. When therapist ratings of Senior Outreach clients ($n = 68$) and of general outpatient clients ($n = 7257$) discharged between April 1980 and June 1981 were compared, it was found that Senior Outreach clients were rated as improved significantly more than general outpatient clients—chi-square $(2) = 33.0$, $p < .01$. For Senior Outreach clients, 43% were rated as improved, 47% as not changed, and 10% as worse. Comparable figures for general outpatient services were 19% improved, 77% not changed, and 4% worse. Unfortunately, data collection at this time did not allow for diagnostic group comparisons, but chapter 11 pursues that question further.

In summary, general evaluation results indicate that clients 60 and over who enter the program seem to be as satisfied with therapy as are younger adults clients, that they are less prone to fail to keep appointments, and they are rated by therapists as showing more improvement. The last finding could be explained as either due to actual higher rates of improvement in the elderly or as due to Senior Outreach therapists being more optimistic in rating change in the elderly than are other therapists in rating change in nonelderly populations. While this distinction is very important and needs further study, at this point in the development of clinical services for the aged and given the extensive speculative literature on therapeutic pessimism about the elderly, either interpretation of this finding is interesting and encouraging. In fact, given the general tone of the literature of mutual aversion, it is somewhat surprising to find that in this program elderly clients and therapists come together and have an experience that is mutually rewarding and may in fact lead to greater therapeutic change than with younger adults.

Program Costs and Income

The issue of costs and income generation are important factors to be considered for any modern program that aspires to more than a brief life as demonstration project. In the Mental Health Department of Ventura County the Senior Outreach program has had a consistently high standing in fiscal management, including procedures such as collection of clients' financial statements, Medi-Cal sticker, and client fees (very few of our clients are ever delinquent). For the first full year of service, the cost of delivering a therapy visit was about 1.5 times that of a regular outpatient clinic. Although it was widely assumed that our productivity per clinician would be lower due to field visits, Senior Outreach staff averaged the same number of client contacts per month as did outpatient clinicians. This would appear to be due to younger adult clients' higher no show rates, to careful planning of home visit routes, and to the use of a four-day week of ten-hour days that increased the number of home visits per work day and so reduced travel time to the office and back. In addition, as of the end of the second year of program operation, the dollar amount of income generated was higher for Senior Outreach than for any other department program.

Goal-Specific Evaluation

As noted earlier, the program was initiated in order to increase the use of outpatient services by the elderly and to prevent unnecessary institutionalization. This section examines program success relative to these specific goals. The addition of new outpatient services does not necessarily lead to an increase in the proportion of elderly in such services. As many therapists, including people who worked with other senior outreach teams that did not offer psychotherapy, argued, one reason for this is that the elderly might not sign up for the outpatient service (i.e., that we would put on a new program and no one would come in). Another reason is that the new program might simply draw elders already being served at other program sites within the Mental Health Department. There was some pressure to encourage such exchanges in the early development of our program, but, as a matter of administrative policy, we maintained that we existed to serve elders who did not otherwise come to our center.

Comparing the period July 1978 to March 1980, when the program started, to April 1980 to December 1981 provides a test that is somewhat biased against the demonstration of program effectiveness since (1) the program manager had been developing a groundwork for senior programs and seeing clients in the October 1979 to March 1980 period, and (2) April 1980 includes start-up time rather than simply operation. Nonetheless, there was an increase in outpatient service utilization by the elderly from 4.7% of adult outpatient clients to 5.6%, a statistically significant increase —chi-square $(1) = 6.33$, $p < .05$. In 1977, when the department began to address underutilization by community education programs, the utilization rate had been only 2%, but in 1981, the percentage of seniors served was 6.4%. In any case, it appears that at the end of eighteen months of operation, the program achieved the goal of increasing the use of outpatient services by the elderly. Follow-up analyses have shown that these gains were maintained at least through 1986 (the last year for which comparable data are available): The percentage of elderly served in outpatient services has remained stable in the 6.5% to 7% range.

Evaluation of success in attaining the second goal, prevention of unnecessary institutionalization of the elderly, has proved more problematic. Institutionalization was initially defined as keeping as many seniors as possible out of the Mental Health Department's inpatient psychiatric unit and of the local state hospital. At first, we intended to achieve this goal by early assessment and intervention with outpatient therapy. We also began the program with an awareness of the danger of increasing institutionalization. There was a tertiary concern with unnecessary nursing home placement. The concern that programs designed to help the elderly often "help" and "protect" them by admitting them to long-term care facilities has been articulated by Zarit (1980) and documented by Nardone (1980). This position, however, involves problems of definition, measurement, and rationale.

In terms of definition, the department's inpatient unit is an acute, short-stay (average stay is less than one week) psychiatric crisis program. This is hardly what one generally conceives of as institutionalization. The state hospital, while more like an institution, offers more active treatment than many long-term care facilities, and, in fact, the depopulation of the geriatric unit there has led to severely disabled elderly being sent to skilled nursing facilities in neighboring counties, often over sixty miles away, which makes it impossible for families (themselves often elderly, ill, and disabled) to visit. For this reason, the reduction of the state hospital geriatric inpatient population from 22 to 7 in a past year was less of a victory than one might expect. In addition, this change was largely due to state and county fiscal policies and was the kind of rerouting referred to by Kahn (1977), not the actual result of treatment intervention.

There is also a problem in rationale—specifically, with the assumption that outpatient therapy is related to inpatient utilization. Most discussions of this issue seem to assume that an increase in outpatient care would yield a decrease in inpatient care—that the usage of the two programs ought to be negatively correlated. However, as we saw in chapter 8, the correlation of inpatient and outpatient utilization by the elderly across counties in California was essentially zero. Looking across time periods rather than across locales, the point-estimate correlation is higher and positive ($r = +.40$) but not significantly different from zero for services in Ventura County in fourteen reporting periods from July 1978 to December 1981. The conclusion would seem to be that use of outpatient therapy and use of inpatient care are unrelated.

However, this conclusion is based on data from programs that do not have an intentionally designed effort to reduce inappropriate use of higher levels of care. The Ventura Program attempted to use outreach outpatient mental health services to reduce clients' needs for institutional levels of care. In the summer of 1982, Deborah Lower-Walker, a medical sociologist, joined the team and assisted us in our efforts to better understand and then to evaluate our charge to reduce unnecessary institutionalization of the elderly. The definitional work was reported by Lower-Walker and myself (1985) and discussed in chapter 1 of this volume. The evaluation is described below.

Study: Reducing Institutionalization of the Elderly

From the outset, we were aware that a major problem in this evaluation was the absence of a control group or even a logical group against which to compare the team's impact on our clients' need for twenty-four-hour care. This flaw makes scientific or even quasi-experimental rigor unattainable. Consequently, we decided to pursue the question by reporting the program's experience and comparing the outcome to the best available estimates of population rates of institutional use. These rates themselves are not well established.

Clients. This study focused on the 33% ($n = 231$) of clients seen for assessment and referral who became outpatient mental health clients of the Senior Outreach Team. These clients were predominantly female (72%), either married (38.5%) or widowed (36.8%) and, like the county, predominantly white (83%). Mean age was 73, with 25% of clients being over 80. All but 17 were living independently at referral. One third were referred by mental health services, 25% by family or friends, and 10% were self-referred. Physical needs included 27.7% having circulatory system disorders. Evaluation and stabilization of medication were needed by 30%. Over 63% had no prior mental health experience. The remainder had previous outpatient therapy (11.3%), crisis contacts (8.7%), or previous state hospital stays (16.5%).

Problems. The initial problems, as defined by the referral source, were classified into the definitions Lower-Walker and I devised (1985) of "at-risk elderly" problem categories. Only 5 out of 231 problems were not classifiable into this schema, which is described in chapter 1. This analysis also reveals the change in definition that can take place in mental health assessment. For example, 6 of 10 with "physical problems" had treatable mental disorders. Of 67 with mental status problems, a category including many "frail" or "confused" problem behaviors, many were seen as depressed (19), psychotic (10), anxious (7), and so forth. Similarly, throughout this study, there was evidence of redefining problems away from frailty due to aging or confusion due to senility and toward treatable (on an outpatient basis) disorders.

Treatment. Treatment included short-term psychotherapy in office and in field settings (60% of cases) as well as psychotropic medication prescribed by the team psychiatrist (28% of cases).

Treatment Outcome. Of 145 cases closed at time of study, 11 clients had died and were excluded from outcome analysis. On the Global Assessment Scale, 55% of clients were rated by therapists as improved, 34% as demonstrating no change, and 11% showed decline. The rating of improvement in terms of the presenting problem is essentially identical. This success rate, while gratifying and replicating results reported earlier in this chapter, is conceptually distinct from preventing unnecessary institutionalization. The following discussion considers the results of outpatient intervention at different levels of institutional care.

Use of Inpatient Mental Health Services. A standard of comparison is difficult to calculate. For the general population of elderly (60+) in California, the 1980 estimate was a 2.2% need for inpatient mental health services. The clients of the outreach team were, of course, defined as "at risk," with 16.5% having previous inpatient stays in state hospitals. Another standard is the ratio of inpatient to outpatient need. This yields 22% of outpatients at risk for psychiatric care. While the general population estimate is almost certainly too low, this "at risk" estimate is certainly too high since many outpatient clients are clearly not at risk of hospitalization. Of Senior Outreach clients, 11.7% were admitted to a short-stay acute inpatient psychiatric unit after initial contact, and 3% went to state hospitals.

Change in Level of Care During Treatment. Again, comparison figures are difficult to obtain. It is generally accepted that at any one time 5% of elders are in institutional care. Lifetime chance of being in a nursing home has been defined as about 25% (Palmore 1976). More recently, McConnel (1984) has argued that even the 25% figure is an underestimate and that lifetime risk is closer to 50%. Weissert and Scanlon (1983) have estimated the rate of frailty and risk of long-term care placement to about 12% for the elderly population as a whole and near 33% for elderly with psychiatric diagnoses. None of these figures is directly comparable to be the population of Senior Outreach clients, and none would present a rigorously defendable estimate of their risk for placement during the time period that they received services.

The team recommended at assessment that 22 people needed residential or higher levels of care. These represent 9.5% of all cases; 2.2% of all cases were recommended for skilled nursing care or psychiatric hospitalization. In fact, by the end of the study, 5 of these individuals were in independent living, changing the actual percentages to 7.4% and 1.3%.

A total of 42 persons moved to residential or higher levels of care while in treatment, the 22 described above, plus 20 who moved without an initial recommendation by Senior Outreach; 18% of all clients were moved into placements, 10% to skilled nursing and psychiatric care.

Were these moves appropriate? Of 19 who moved into residential care placements, 6 were memory impaired, 6 chronically mentally ill, and 5 severely depressed. Of 16 who moved to skilled nursing, 5 were demented, 3 psychotic, and 7 severely depressed. Fourteen elders in this latter group suffered increased physical deterioration prior to the move.

Who decided the move? In the two instances of referral to locked skilled nursing care, the team made the referral after several unlocked board and care placements had been terminated by the facilities. Acute inpatient staff made the five referrals to state hospital, and Senior Outreach made the initial admission. Table 9.1 shows the numbers placed by the person(s)

TABLE 9.1: Placement Decisions by Level of Care

	Residential Care	Skilled Nursing	Total
Senior Outreach Recommended	8	6	14
Patient Decided	7	2	9
Third Party Decided	4	8	12
	19	16	35

making the placement referral decision. At both residential and skilled nursing levels, the majority of such decisions were made without the involvement of Senior Outreach. (In the skilled nursing instance, the third parties were families and hospitals, often in combination.) This finding underscores the fact that teams such as ours can only advise about alternatives; the power to decide is elsewhere.

Conclusion. With only very rough population standards for comparison, it is difficult to evaluate the impact of the team on prevention of inappropriate institutionalization for this group judged at risk. In my judgment, the team was successful in that rates of use of institutional care were lower than might be expected from available crude predictors and because those who moved were both mentally and (in the skilled nursing facility level) physically frail.

Future directions of investigation should include:

1. Attempts to define the "at risk" group in a measurable way at the population level and to determine rates of institutionalization of this group under varying resource conditions;

2. Further attempts to demonstrate the value of treatment oriented versus supportive and "case management only" types of care in prevention of inappropriate institutionalization; and

3. Exploration of circumstances under which elders themselves choose higher levels of care.

CONCLUSIONS AND IMPLICATIONS

The Senior Outreach Program was designed to meet the twin goals of increasing the accessibility of outpatient services and prevention of unnecessary institutionalization. With regard to addressing the underutilization of services, this program began with a rationale concerning the mutual aversion of therapists and the aged, instituted a program based on that rationale, and has met with some success.

With regard to our second goal, while originally we accepted the assumption that early outpatient intervention is effective enough to prevent institutionalization, we now have reached something of a quandary in understanding and measuring this goal. Our very rudimentary attempt to address the issue is, to my knowledge, the only data now available on the impact of outpatient mental health services on institutionalization. Although this data may provide some basis for cautious optimism, research that tests program effectiveness against logically chosen comparison groups is clearly needed. Our experience raises more questions than it provides answers.

1. What, in fact, is the range of institutionalization? There is considerable variation in programs and in quality of care among psychiatric units, state hospitals, and nursing homes. In specific instances, higher levels of care feel less institutional than lower levels and appear more humane than some families' attempts at home care.

2. Whatever does constitute *appropriate* institutionalization is a complex match of client need and available services. Far too many deinstitutionalization and prevention programs work with elders who are in no danger of being institutionalized (see Weissert, Wan, and Liveriatos 1980). At the same time, programs sometimes advocate that no one should be institutionalized, although logic and experience suggest that for some elderly twenty-four-hour care must be the most humane available alternative.

3. Many programs seem to direct the frail and severely disabled elder from one dreary setting to another. Very few programs (the one reported by Penner, Eberly, and Patterson [1983] is an exception) have even a theory as to why their approach ought to work, much less a demonstration of effectiveness.

4. The very frail and disabled elderly have become a political and fiscal hot potato being tossed from one system to another because they are seen as untreatable and very expensive. The problem is likely to continue unless therapeutic nihilism is effectively challenged and program costs are held down and/or allocated in some rational way. This will only take place if

researchers, clinicians, and policy makers all collaborate to address this problem.

This study has reported data that supports the concept that the outreach methods of the mobile geriatric team worked to increase the percentage of older adults seen in outpatient clinics at the mental health department and that the older adults seen for outpatient therapy benefitted from it. It also demonstrates some suggestive evidence that the team had a positive impact on reducing unnecessary institutionalization in a high risk group. The next chapter extends the evaluation to the team's outreach efforts to minority group elderly.

10

Outreach to Hispanic Elderly

As has been discussed in earlier chapters, outreach methods in community mental health have been developed for a variety of underserved populations including low-income persons and members of various minority groups. While the elderly are often considered an underserved population, it is important that this designation for the elderly in general not be allowed to obscure the fact that there are subgroups of older people with special needs, including older members of racial and ethnic minority groups.

Within the population of the aged, it is recognized that certain subgroups, especially minorities, suffer from the "double jeopardy" of being old and minorities (Butler and Lewis 1977; National Urban League 1964). This layering of barriers between the minority elderly and mental health services poses two categories of questions: Will outreach methods developed for providing services to the elderly in general prove effective with minority group elderly? Are there culturally specific changes in such methods that will need to be made with each subpopulation?

This chapter describes an extension of outreach methods developed for the elderly in general to one minority group, the Hispanic (mostly Mexican-American) elderly of Ventura County, California. The evaluation of one program's effectiveness with one population of minority elderly provides an important first step toward understanding the barriers to one minority group's receiving mental health services and ways in which those barriers may be removed.

Are Senior Outreach methods also usable with minority populations? The principal minority group in Ventura County are Hispanics, who comprise 22% of the total population and 9.8% of the population age 60 and over. Hispanics are also the second largest minority group in the United States. The waves of immigration into Southern California imply the existence of groups of Hispanics at several levels of acculturation, between the recently arrived Mexican immigrant to native-born, fully acculturated Mexican-Americans with three or more generations of ancestors born in the United States (Cortese 1979). Work with Hispanic clients requires facility in Spanish as well as an understanding of cultural differences (Lacayo 1980; Cortese 1979). Mexican Americans are often portrayed as having an unsophisticated relationship to the medical system in general and to mental health in particular and as relying instead on the folk medicine of the *curanderos* (folkhealers) (Cuellar 1981). There is often a strong supposition that all Hispanics and especially the Hispanic elderly avoid formal service systems and prefer to "take care of their own."

There is reason to question these views, however. Iverson (1982) describes the use of medical services by Hispanics as greater dependence on *sobadoros* (cure by massage, not unlike chiropractors in Anglo culture) and the continuing use of the Mexican medical system, described as more personal, more dependent on interview than on invasive lab techniques, and less likely to require the patient to undress regardless of presenting problem. Barrera (1982) reviews the literature on mental health services to Hispanics of all ages and concludes that Hispanics utilize mental health services as much as or more than Anglos. Finally, some studies suggest that Hispanics see a greater role for the government in service provision than do Anglos (see Lacayo 1980).

This mix of presumed problems and impressions led to the adoption of an experimental attitude on the part of the Senior Outreach Program. In 1981 a Spanish-speaking mental health nurse with several years experience in crisis intervention was added to the program. The beginning supposition was that we would provide the same pattern of outreach services to the Hispanic elderly as had been provided to non-Hispanic elderly and adapt services as necessary. The Senior Outreach model of community education, assessment, and outpatient therapy was extended to the Spanish-speaking elderly.

EXPERIMENT

Method

Participants. The subjects for the study were the following four groups: (1) 144 Hispanic elderly seen by the Senior Outreach Program between March 1980 and November 1984 for assessment and referral services; (2) 1,320 non-Hispanic elderly seen during that same period for assessment and referral; (3) 39 Hispanics who continued with the Senior Outreach Program in individual psychotherapy, often delivered in the client's home; and (4) 469 non-Hispanics who continued in outpatient psychotherapy.

Measures. The measures include: (1) percentage of each group (Hispanic and non-Hispanic) seen for assessment and referral; (2) percentage of each group seen for outpatient psychotherapy; (3) percentage of each group making the transition from assessment interview to therapy; and (4) change in Global Assessment Scale (GAS) rating, a global measure of client functioning taken by the therapist before and after therapy (Spitzer, Gibbon, and Endicott 1976). In addition, the Hispanic and non-Hispanic groups were compared in terms of readily observed demographic variables and sources of referral to the Senior Outreach Program.

Design. The departure of the Spanish-speaking nurse for advanced training for six months in 1984 provided an opportunity for a "naturally occuring experiment" using a quasi-experimental ABAB design for evaluation of this program. Data collected prior to her hiring form the first baseline (A1); the time from hiring to her leaving for training is the first treatment period (B1); her absence for training provides a "return to baseline" period (A2); and her return to work checks for a return to the intervention level (B2). Post hoc comparisons of other demographic characteristics (gender, age, marital status, and referral source) provide a rough preliminary check of possible competing explanations for observed differences in service utilization.

Results

The results for the assessment visits show that the percentage of Hispanic elderly seen during A1 was 6.8% and rapidly rose to 10.7% during B1, a level that is slightly higher than the percentage of Hispanics in the local population of the elderly. During A2, the percentage fell to 7.0%, relative to the baseline level, and at B2, it rose again to the B1 level of 11%. A similar pattern is seen for those persons receiving outpatient mental health services, with no Hispanics seen during A1, 9.5% during B1, a fall to 7.8% during A2, and an increase back to 11.3% during B2. The percentage of persons making the transition from assessment visit to ongoing therapy is also an important measure of the outreach effort. For the total time period, the percentage of Hispanics making this transition was 27%, which is significantly less than the non-Hispanic percentage of 35.5%— $z = 2.03, p < .05$. However, with the exclusion of cases opened during A1 and A2, the figures change to 33% and 34.7%, which are not significantly different— $z = 0.66$. In other words, the presence of a bilingual-bicultural worker eliminated the difference between Hispanics and non-Hispanics in the percentage of persons assessed who stayed with the program for therapeutic intervention.

Chi-square comparisons of clients seen for assessment visits reveal significant differences between Hispanic and non-Hispanic clients for gender $X = 4.66$, $p < .05$; age, $X = 9.96, p < .05$; and for referral source $X = 22.6$, $p < .01$; but not for marital status. Post hoc analysis shows that a higher proportion of referrals of Hispanic clients were male. The age difference post hoc analysis showed more Hispanics in their 60s and fewer in their 90s. Post hoc procedures show that the difference for referral source was due to fewer Hispanics being referred by crisis-oriented mental health services and more being referred by generic social services, such as the welfare department caseworkers.

For Hispanic clients entering therapy and terminating before this evaluation ($N = 34$), the average change in GAS rating was 6.53 ($s = 12.6$). For the period for which there were data on a comparable group of Anglos (March 1983 to February 1984), the Hispanic mean was 3.25 and the Anglo mean 6.30, a nonsignificant difference—$t = 1.02$.

Discussion

The ABAB design provides considerable credibility to the idea that what was done worked well. The failure to have a complete return to baseline reflects the increased commitment of the whole team to this population with all clinicians seeing some Hispanics who speak English well and the team psychiatrist having learned some Spanish in order to continue services.

The question of what was done can only by answered in a global and impressionistic way since process measures were not taken. The major change was the addition of Spanish language capability to the Senior Outreach method, which thus receives a test of replicability of Senior Outreach methods by extension to a different subgroup. Cultural changes appear to have been relatively minor: There was some need to be respectful of those natural helpgivers in the environment (called *servidores* by Valle and Martinez 1981) who function much like social workers except that they are unpaid. There was also a recognition of the need that clients had to occasionally give small gifts (oranges from a tree in the yard) to the visiting therapist to maintain politeness and respect. The assessment process was altered in that the Kahn Mental Status Questionnaire, translated into Spanish, was often used as a guideline, but questions about family structure, recent community events, and the happenings in *telenovelas* (similar to soap operas) were used as a supplement. The inability to remember U.S. presidents was given less weight in these evaluations than were inabilities to get family relationships correct. Psychotherapy and family sessions were not greatly different in our experience, but this conclusion should be tempered by the observation that our bicultural therapist could have made alterations without being acutely aware of them.

Our impression is that, if anything, those Hispanic elderly with recent ties to Mexico are more open to therapy than are either Anglos or the more acculturated Mexican-American. This observation, of course, needs empirical verification, but it is consistent with Barrera's (1982) conclusions about Hispanics of all ages. This tentative conclusion does differ sharply from the pessimism implied by the "double jeopardy" concept.

The observed sex difference probably reflects the greater proportion of men among the Hispanic elderly in the county (47% compared to 43%). Similarly, the age difference probably reflects population differences: among non-Hispanic elderly (60+), 26% are over 75 in this county; among Hispanics, only 22% are over 75. The referral source differences confirm the relative inaccessibility of mental health services, even crisis-oriented ones, and a greater presence of Hispanic elders and a willingness to refer them in the formal social service system, with comparable referrals from all other sources.

Finally, the absence of a difference in therapist-rated change in the Hispanic elderly as compared to Anglo elderly is promising, though far from conclusive, in terms of the effects of therapy on this often overlooked group of potential users of mental health services.

SUMMARY

In terms of designing interventions for "double jeopardy" populations, the current study provides data for an optimistic response. One such population, the Hispanic (mostly Mexican-American) elderly of an urban southern California community were found to be receptive to outreach methods designed for majority group elderly and adapted mainly by use of Spanish-speaking staff and with little conscious change for cultural factors. Generalizability to other populations must be cautious and based on further research. Mexican-American elderly of the rural Southwest may require different methods. Puerto Rican elderly in the urban Northeast probably require different types of adaptation. Certainly, there are likely to be differences in application to black elderly and for Asian American elderly. These results do, however, provide a basis for challenging the often heard and too little examined assumption that minority group elderly "take care of their own" and would not want our services even if we did take the trouble to make them available. Our experience stands in sharp contrast and found this population ready and eager to use our services if they were made physically and linguistically accessible.

These last two chapters have reported results of evaluation studies that support a spirit of optimism in providing psychotherapy to older adults, both Anglos and Hispanic. The next chapter goes beyond this finding of effectiveness to explore the factors contributing to successful outcomes within the older population.

11

Factors Influencing Therapy Outcome with the Elderly

While the evaluations of therapeutic outcome reported in the previous chapters were positive and encouraging about the ability of older clients to benefit from outpatient mental health treatment, it would be of interest to compare the affects of age on therapy outcome to other factors that might be expected to influence outcome in psychotherapy.

In Chapter 9, it was established that early on in the mobile geriatric outreach program therapist-rated change was greater for older clients as compared to younger adult clients in outpatient clinics at the same center. The result leaves numerous questions unanswered: Will this greater improvement of older adults be stable over time or will it prove to be the result of early enthusiasm yielding large results in a novel program? How does age compare to other variables that might affect therapist-rated change? For example, is gender more important in determining therapy outcome than client age? Schlossberg (1984) summarizes other areas in social gerontology where gender is a more important determinant than age.

Other client characteristics may be expected to have an impact on treatment outcome as well. In therapeutic work with older persons, an often neglected client variable is psychological diagnosis. Settin (1982) clearly demonstrated that clinicians often confound diagnosis and age, being more willing to label a client as suffering from organic disorders and psychosis when the client is identified as being older. Older persons may have higher rates of organic disorders, but the vast majority are not organically impaired, and diagnosis both differs conceptually from chronological age and deserves consideration as a potential explanation of variation in treatment outcome among older people.

Oddly, there has been little attention to the effects of process variables in outcome of mental health interventions with the elderly. Will therapist assignment, number of sessions, and type of treatment (e.g., medication versus psychotherapy) make a difference in outcome of outpatient therapy with the elderly? If there are age effects in outcome among the elderly, can these be modified by altering process in therapy?

This chapter reports a follow-up evaluation of the Senior Outreach

Program's effectiveness with older adults (age 60 and over). The reliability of the earlier results is checked by replication with a new sample of clients seen two years after the original study. The comparison to younger adults is replicated both by percentage reporting change and by comparison of mean levels of change. Within the sample of older adults, multivariate analyses are used to measure and compare the relative influence of chronological age, other client variables including functional status and diagnosis, and treatment variables on therapist-rated change in therapy.

EXPERIMENT

Method

Participants. The principal group of subjects for this study were the 125 clients of Senior Outreach who terminated therapy between March 1983 and February 1984. Clients were recruited by outreach methods, and about 50% of therapy visits took place in the client's home or in other field settings; the other visits were clinic visits. Female clients numbered 77%. The age range was from 60 to 94, and the average age was 72. In this group, 73% had at least one physical disorder, with the most common classes of illness being circulatory disorders, neurological problems, endocrine disorders, and cancers. Psychological disorders as assessed by the admitting clinicians included adjustment disorders (44%), affective disorders (28%), organic brain syndrome disorders (8.8%), psychoses (7.9%), and anxiety states (7.1%). The remaining clients had a variety of diagnoses including psychosomatic disorders, sexual dysfunction, and disorders of impulse control.

In addition, for comparison of change in therapy, the following groups were used: (1) 68 older persons seen at Senior Outreach between April 1980 and June 1981; (2) 7,257 adults age 18–64 seen in all Ventura County Mental Health Outpatient Clinics in 1980–1981; (3) 135 older adults seen at Senior Outreach between March 1980 and June 1982; and (4) 1,181 adults age 18–64 seen at Ventura city and vicinity community mental health clinics in 1983–1984. The first three groups are previously reported (Knight 1983; and Lower and Knight 1983). The two comparison groups of elderly clients are overlapping and are used because for historical reasons, the first sample was analyzed using percentage of clients reporting change, while the second used mean change for older clients.

At the time of this study, the therapists included two mental health nurses, a clinical social worker, a clinical psychologist, and a psychiatrist. The general therapy orientation was eclectic, but it did have a brief,

Integrating Research and Practice

problem-oriented focus. Some clients received only psychotherapy (56%), some only psychotropic medications (8%), and others a combination (28%). The remainder received only an assessment.

Measures. The measures used in this evaluation were archival data from the problem-oriented record system maintained by Ventura County Mental Health Services. These included: therapist, sex of client, and age of client; diagnosis (DSM III, recoded into categories of organic brain syndrome, psychosis, affective disorder, anxiety disorders, adjustment reactions, and other disorders; in correlational analyses, these categories, as listed above, were numbered from 1 to 6, descending in degree of severity), number of sessions, and type of treatment (psychotherapy only, medication only, therapy and medication, assessment only); illness recorded as none reported, diagnosis deferred, and illness reported; and Global Assessment Scale (GAS) rating (Spitzer, Gibbon, and Endicott 1976) at admission and at discharge as rated by clinician. GAS change is calculated by subtracting GAS at admission from GAS at discharge.

Design. The study is designed as a retrospective program evaluation and as such has certain strengths, including enhanced generalizability based on greater similarity to field conditions (in that therapists and clients control the type, nature, and length of therapy), the nonobtrusive nature of the measures, and the use of true clinical cases as subjects. Findings regarding differential treatment effectiveness between comparison groups and differential impact of client and treatment variables will, of course, need further verification in more highly controlled research environments that permit randomized designs and more precise measurement.

Results

In analysis of the replicability of the outcome results, GAS change from one GAS category (ten-point ranges) to the next has been stable from 1980–1981 to 1983–1984 for the two distinct samples of older clients. Mean levels have also been stable as compared to a 1980–1982 period analyzed by Lower and Knight (1983). For this sample, the mean GAS change is 5.83, as compared to 7.63 in the Lower and Knight sample—$t = 1.46$, N.S.

In comparison to an adult population in community mental health, the Senior Outreach sample showed that a higher percentage of clients improved relative to the percentage of clients changing from one ten-point block to the next—$X = 12.3$, $p < .01$—and in comparison of mean change scores—$t = 3.27$, $p < .01$. In short, both the degree of change and the supeiority to reported change in younger adult samples was maintained from the beginning of the program to three years later with different clients.

Since the major outcome variable is therapist-rated outcome, therapist differences on other variables are of interest in interpreting therapist-rated outcome. Therapists show significant differences in GAS rating at admission—F (4,120) = 5.16, p < .001—and on illness of client—$X^2 = 17.21$, $p < .02$. Therapist effect on psychological diagnosis could not be assessed due to a high percentage of cell frequencies less than 5. An examination of ratings and patient illness by therapist indicates that two team members, the psychiatrist and the mental health nurse doing outreach to Hispanic elderly, had clients with lower initial global functioning and with more physical illness. While it is clearly possible that this reflects some therapist bias in rating, it is also clear that these two team members tended to work with more impaired and more physically ill clients.

Contributing Factors: Multivariate Analysis. In order to assess the contribution of the various measured variables to change in GAS rating during therapy, a multiple regression analysis was performed. First, all variables were entered, and then those with apparently small contributions to explained variance were deleted, with F tests performed to test for significant decreases in amount of explained variance. The procedure is essentially a post hoc "step down" multiple regression to generate a model to explain observed data rather than a hypothesis-testing analysis. GAS at admission was not entered in the equation since a negative relationship of GAS change to GAS at admission will usually be obtained and is essentially a statistical artifact. Age and number of sessions in therapy emerge as the major predictors of outcome with a multiple correlation of .24 $(F = 3.63, p < .05)$ explaining 6% of the variance. Age and number of session are equal in relative strength, with age being negatively related to therapist rated-change and number of sessions in therapy being positively related. Post hoc examination of mean scores shows that the oldest clients (those over 80) gain the most from longer sessions of therapy, improving as much as do the younger elderly clients in brief therapy (see Table 11.1).

Another statistical method for considering outcome in therapy is the analysis of the GAS score at the end of therapy. Using the step down regression analysis, four factors are found to account for 50% of the variance in final GAS rating. These are age, number of sessions in therapy, GAS at beginning of therapy, and diagnosis. However, once again, GAS at beginning of therapy must be considered conceptually suspect. Even though it accounts for much of the effect, the fact that those who are functionally better before therapy are also functionally better at the end is of little

TABLE 11.1: Effects of Age
and Number of Sessions
in Therapy on Change

Age	Number of Sessions		
	<8	8–16	>16
60–69	4.07	11.54	10.62
70–79	5.67	6.00	7.31
80+	−4.44	3.00	6.55

interest. Deleting GAS at admission also minimizes the importance of age and number of sessions in therapy, leaving diagnosis coded as a dummy variable explaining 24% of the variance. However, since diagnosis is a categorical variable and is itself correlated with GAS at admission, an analysis of covariance using GAS at admission as the covariate is a more appropriate statistical analysis. In this analysis of covariance, diagnosis remains significant—F (5, 118) = 3.62, $p < .01$—and accounted for 10% of the variance, with functional level at admission held constant statistically and accounting for 25% of the variance. A post hoc examination of mean scores suggests that persons with psychoses and anxiety states show the greatest change in treatment, while those with depression and adjustment disorders show more modest change and those with organic disorders show no change.

Discussion

The present study replicates earlier findings that therapy with the elderly has positive results as measured by therapist-rated change in global functioning. The changes remain higher than change in younger adult populations receiving outpatient therapy in community mental health. These results, while far from conclusive, are certainly encouraging. Future studies are needed to confirm these results with client-rated change scores as well as ratings by significant others and more structured measures of change.

Given that change occurs, it is interesting to seek factors that mediate or explain that change. In the analysis of change scores, age and number of sessions in therapy influenced these scores, with age in the over-60 group showing a negative effect on therapeutic change and number of sessions in therapy having a positive effect. Post hoc analysis suggests that these opposing effects can balance one another such that older clients who have more therapy sessions change as much as younger elderly with fewer sessions. Clearly, this finding requires further study in which persons of different age levels are assigned to various lengths of therapy. It would also be valuable to assess other factors, such as functional status and health, independently of the outcome measure in order to better understand the age effect found here.

The analysis of final ratings of functioning identifies diagnosis alone as the principal effect, retaining much of its predictive power even when functional level at admission to therapy is held constant. This suggests a major role in prediction of therapeutic outcome for a client variable other than age, a variable that is conceptually central to predicting therapeutic outcome at any age. Again, it is clearly necessary to do controlled experimental studies with planned control of functional level within diagnostic groups to further support this observation.

Aside from confirming the value of mental health treatment for older persons with psychological disorders, the current study illustrates the complex role of age as a variable influencing therapy-rated change. Those over 60 are seen to improve more than younger adults. Within the over-60 group, age emerges as a negative influence on change but as equivalent in strength to time in therapy and possibly offset by longer courses of therapy for the very old (those over 80). Further research with more precise measures of functional status, therapeutic process variables, and the underlying variables that are crudely captured by chronological age is clearly needed to extend our understanding of therapeutic change in older adults.

SUMMARY

This chapter serves to substantiate more completely that older adults do benefit from outpatient mental health services—from psychotherapy and psychotropic medication, both separately and in combination. The most surprising result is that they benefit more than younger adults seen at other clinics of the same department of mental health. This finding raises more questions than the limited data of this study can answer. For example, did the younger adults differ diagnostically? Were they in some sense more seriously and chronically disabled than the elderly who were seen. These are important questions, and they deserve to be studied by further better designed research. Over a decade ago, the question to be discussed was "Can any older adult benefit from therapy?" That this question has changed to "Why do older adults appear to benefit more than younger ones from these community mental health interventions?" is significant.

Afterword: Lessons from the Ventura Team's Experience

This book has described a model of outreach to the elderly based on an understanding of the elderly's different need for mental health services, the role of mental disorder in frailty among the elderly, the position of mental health services in the range of services for the aged, and barriers to mental health services for the elderly, with the latter being addressed through an educational approach that includes both educating the elderly about psychological problems and educating the community about mental health services and their role in improving the lives of older people. The development of the Ventura Senior Outreach Team was discussed in relation to these principles with special attention to the history of the decision to offer psychotherapy to the elderly and to the use of this double educational approach.

Assessment, therapy, and educational issues were discussed in more detail, with particular attention given to changes required by working with the elderly and changes that arise when delivering services in the home setting. A model of services to the demented elderly and their families, which clarifies the potential contribution of mental health services to what is often incorrectly seen as an insoluble problem, is presented The emotional hazards of outreach work with the elderly are discussed with a view to preparing persons coming to work in this area more thoroughly for the challenges that geriatric outreach can present.

A research program addressing a variety of issues was described. It suggested a need for a change of focus in barriers to therapy research from therapist bias to systems-level barriers, documented the effectiveness of this program in increasing utilization of outpatient therapy, indicated that older people not only benefit from outpatient therapy but do so to a greater degree than younger adult mental health center clients; it also explored factors affecting therapeutic outcome, and evaluated the extension of mental health services to the Hispanic elderly.

Are there essential ingredients of this approach? I believe that educating the elderly about psychological problems and demystifying mental health services for the elderly, their families, aging services workers, and mental health professionals are essential parts of outreach. Furthermore, it would appear impossible to provide services to this population without doing home visits and without some way to reduce fees below usual private practice levels. These last have important policy implications in that Medicare and Medicaid and many private insurers tend to discourage home visits and provide minimal coverage for outpatient mental health services.

Can this approach work elsewhere? Many people have expressed the opinion that there must be something unique about Ventura County for this program to have worked. My own evaluation is that the primary unique element was the willingness to attempt the program when it was tried. In general, everything has worked out more easily and we have achieved better results than we expected. I can only encourage others to try such work with the same spirit of cautious optimism about mental health work with the elderly. At this time, it would appear that while those who have not tried to provide mental health services to the elderly believe that such services are not likely to be effective, those who have worked with the elderly have found it easier than they expected, and they have found the work rewarding as well.

References

Barrera, M. 1982. Raza populations. In L. R. Snowden, ed., *Reaching the underserved*. Beverly Hills: Sage.

Bekker, R. A., and C. Taylor. 1966. Attitudes toward the aged in a multigenerational sample. *Journal of Gerontology* 21:115–18.

Bennett, R., and J. Eckman. 1973. Attitudes toward aging: A critical examination of recent literature. In C. Eisdorfer and M. P. Lawton, eds., *Psychology of adult development and aging*. Washington, D. C.: American Psychological Association.

Blazer, D., D. C. Hughes, and L. K. George. 1987. The epidemiology of depression in an elderly community population. *Gerontologist* 27:281–87.

Blenkner, M., M. Bloom, and M. A. Nielson. 1971. A research and demonstration project of protective services. *Social Casework* 52:488–99.

Blumenthal, M. November 1980. Mental deterioration and family burden. Paper presented at the meeting of the Gerontological Society of America, San Diego.

Broskowski, A. 1976. Management information systems for planning and evaluation. In H. C. Schulberg, ed., *Program evaluation in the health fields*. New York: Behavioral Publications.

Brothwood, J. 1971. The organization and development of services for the aged with special reference to the mentally ill. In D. W. K. Kay and A. Walk, eds., *Recent developments in psychogeriatrics*. Ashford (Kent), England: Headley Bros.

Butler, R. N., and M. I. Lewis. 1977. *Aging and mental health*. St. Louis: Mosby.

Campbell, D. T., and D. W. Fiske. 1959. Convergent and discriminant validation by the multitrait-multimethod matrix. *Psychological Bulletin* 56:81–105.

Cichetti, D. V., C. R. Fletcher, E. Lerner, and J. F. Coleman. 1973. Effects of a social medicine course on the attitudes of medical students toward the elderly. *Journal of Gerontology* 28:370–73.

Coe, R.M. 1967. Professional perspectives on the aged. *Gerontologist* 7:114–19.

Cortese, M. 1979. Intervention research with Hispanic Americans: A review. *Hispanic Journal of Behavioral Sciences* 1:4–20.

Craik, F. I. M., and S. Trehub. 1982. *Aging and cognitive processes*. New York: Plenum.

Cuellar, I. 1981. Service delivery and mental health services for Chicano elderly. In M. Miranda and R. A. Ruiz, eds., *Chicago aging and mental health*. Department of Health and Human Services Pub. No. ADM 81–952. Washington, D.C.: Government Printing Office.

Dye, C. J. 1978. Psychologists' role in the provision of mental health care for the elderly. *Professional Psychology* 9:38–49.

Eisdorfer, C., and J. Altrocchi. 1961. A comparison of attitudes toward old age and mental illness. *Journal of Gerontology* 16:340–43.

Essex, D. September 1981. *Client satisfaction survey.* Ventura County Mental Health Memorandum.

Essex, D. April 1982. *No show rates and scheduling procedures.* Ventura County Mental Health Memorandum.

Estes, C. 1979. *The aging enterprise.* San Francisco: Jossey-Bass.

Fiore, J., J. Becker, and D. B. Coppel. 1983. Social network interactions: A buffer or a stress? *American Journal of Community Psychology* 11:423–39.

Fleming A. S., L. D. Richards, J. F. Santos, and P. R. West. 1986. *Mental health services for the elderly,* vol. 3. Washington, D.C.: Retirement Research Foundation.

Folstein M., J. C. Anthony, I. Parhad, B. Duffy, and E. M. Gruenberg. 1985. The meaning of cognitive impairment in the elderly. *Journal of American Geriatrics Society.* 33:228–35.

Folstein, M. F., S. E. Folstein, and P. R. McHugh. 1975. "Mini-mental state": A practical method for grading the cognitive state of patients for the clinician. *Journal of Psychiatric Research* 12:189–98.

Frankfather, D. 1977. *The aged in the community.* New York: Praeger.

Garfield, S. L. 1978. Research on client variables in psychotherapy. In S. L. Garfield and A. E. Bergin, eds., *Handbook of psychotherapy and behavior change.* New York: John Wiley.

Gartner, A., and F. Riesman, eds. 1984. *The self-help revolution.* New York: Human Sciences.

Gatz, M., S. J. Popkin, C. D. Pino, and G. R. VanderBor. 1985. Psychological interventions with older adults. In J. E. Birren and K. W. Schaie, eds., *Handbook of psychology and aging.* New York: Van Nostrand.

Gatz, M., M. A. Smyer, and M. P. Lawton. 1980. The mental health system and the older adult. In L. W. Poon, ed., *Aging in the 1980's: Psychological issues.* Washington, D.C.: American Psychological Association.

General Accounting Office. 1982. *The elderly remain in need of mental health services.* Pub. no. GAO/HRD 82–112. Washington, D.C.: Government Printing Office.

Goldfarb, A. I., and J. Sheps. 1954. Psychotherapy of the aged. *Psychosomatic Medicine* 16.

Gray, V. K. 1983. Providing support for home care givers. In M. A. Smyer and M. Gatz, eds., *Mental health and aging: Programs and evaluations.* Beverly Hills: Sage.

Gurin, G., J. Veroff, and S. Feld. 1960. *Americans view their mental health.* New York: Basic Books.

Gurland, B., R. R. Golden, J. A. Teresi, and J. Challop. 1984. The SHORT-CARE: An efficient instrument for the assessment of depression, dementia, and disability. *Journal of Gerontology* 39:166–69.

Haley, W. E., E. C. Levine, S. L. Brown, J. W. Berry, and G. H. Hughes. 1987. Psychological, social and health consequences of caring for relatives with senile dementia. *Journal of the American Geriatrics Society* 35:405–11.

Harris, L., and Associates. 1975. *The myth and reality of aging in America.* Washington, D.C.: National Council on Aging.

Iverson, E. June 1982. Accessibility of health services for Mexican Americans. Paper presented at the meeting of the Pacific Division of the American Association for the Advancement of Science, Santa Barbara, Calif.

Kahn, R. 1977. Perspectives in the evaluation of psychological mental health programs for the aged. In W. D. Gentry, ed., *Geropsychology. A model of training and clinical service.* Cambridge, Mass.: Ballinger.

Kastenbaum, R. 1964. The reluctant therapist. In R. Kastenbaum, ed., *New thoughts on old age.* New York: Springer.

Kastenbaum, R. 1978. Personality theory. Therapeutic Approaches and the elderly. In M. Storandt, I. C. Siegler, and M. F. Elias, eds. *The clinical psychology of aging.* New York: Plenum.

Kay, D. W. K., and K. Bergmann. 1980. Epidemiology of mental disorders among the aged in the community. In J. E. Birren and R. B. Sloane, eds., *Handbook of mental health and aging,* Englewood Cliffs, N. J.: Prentice Hall.

Kintsch, W. 1970. *Learning, memory, and conceptual processes.* New York: John Wiley.

Klatsky, R. L. 1975. *Human memory.* San Francisco: Freeman.

Knee, R., and G. Krueger. 1981. *Resource guide for mental health and support services for the elderly.* Department of Health and Human Services Pub. No. ADM81–985. Washington, D.C.: Government Printing Office.

Knight, B. G. 1978–1979. Psychotherapy and behavior change with the non-institutionalized aged. *International Journal of Aging and Human Development* 9:221–36.

Knight, B. G. April 1981. Never too late: A role induction film. Media Festival presentation at the meeting of the Western Gerontological Society, Seattle.

Knight, B. G. 1983. Assessing a mobile outreach team. In M. A. Smyer and M. Gatz, eds., *Mental health and aging: Programs and evaluations.* Beverly Hills: Sage.

Knight, B. G. 1986a. *Psychotherapy with the older adult.* Beverly Hills: Sage.

Knight, B. G. 1986b. Therapists' attitudes as explanation of Underservice of elderly in mental health: Testing an old hypothesis. *International Journal of Aging and Human Development* 22:261–69.

Knight, B. G., and D. Lower-Walker. 1985. Toward a definition of alternatives to institutionalization for the frail elderly. *Gerontologist* 25:358–63.

Knight, B. G., R. A. Reinhart, and P. Field. 1982. Senior outreach services: A treatment-oriented outreach team in community mental health. *Gerontologist* 22:544–47.

Knight, B. G., R. W. Wollert, L. H. Levy, C. L. Frame, and V. Padgett. 1980. Self-help groups: The members' perspectives. *American Journal of Community Psychology* 8:53–65.

Kogan, N. 1961. Attitude toward older people: The development of a scale and an examination of correlates. *Journal of Abnormal and Social Psychology* 62:44–45.

Kogan, N., and M. A. Wallach. 1961. Age changes in values and attitudes. *Journal of Gerontology* 16:340–43.

Kubler-Ross, E. 1969. *On death and dying.* New York: Macmillan.

Lacayo, C. G. 1980. *A national study to assess the service needs of the Hispanic elderly.* Los Angeles: Associacion Nacional pro Personas Mayores.

LaRue, A., C. Dessonville, and L. Jarvik. 1985. Aging and mental disorders. In J. E. Birren and K. W. Schaie, eds., *Handbook of psychology and aging.* New York: Van Nostrand.

Levy, L. H. 1978. Professionals' view of self-help groups. *American Journal of Community Psychology* 6:305–13.

Little, A. D. 1976. *A working manual of simple program evaluation techniques for community mental health centers.* Department of Health, Education, and Welfare Pub. No. (Adm), 76–404. Washington, D.C.: Government Printing Office.

Lower, D. L., and B. G. Knight. November 1983. The geriatric mental health outreach team as an alternative to institutionalization. In B. Knight. (chair), Treatment oriented approaches to prevention of institutionalization. Symposium at the meeting of the Gerontological Society of America, San Francisco.

Mace, N., and P. Rabins. 1981. *The 36 hour day.* Baltimore: Johns Hopkins University Press.

Mattis, S. 1976. Mental status examination for organic mental syndrome. In R. Bellack and B. Karasu, eds., *Geriatric psychiatry.* New York: Grune and Stratton.

McConnel, C. E. 1984. A note on the lifetime risk of nursing home residency. *Gerontologist* 24:193–98.

McTavish, D. G. 1971. Perceptions of older people. *Gerontologist* 11:90–101.

Morycz, R. K. 1980. An exploration of senile dementia and family burden. *Clinical Social Work Journal* 8:16–27.

Myers, J. K., and Associates. 1984. Six month prevalence of psychiatric disorders in three communities. *Archives of General Psychiatry* 41:959–67.

Nardi, A. H. 1973. Person perception research and the perception of life span development. In P. B. Baltes and K. W. Schaie, eds., *Life span developmental psychology.* New York: Academic Press.

Nardone, M. 1980. Characteristics predicting community care for mentally impaired older persons. *Gerontologist* 20:660–68.

National Urban League. 1964. *Double jeopardy: The older Negro in America.* New York: National Urban League.

Neugarten, B. L., and G. O. Hagestad. 1976. Age and the life course. In R. H. Binstock and E. Shanas, eds., *Handbook of aging and the social sciences.* New York: Van Nostrand.

Niederehe G. 1986. Depression and memory impairment in the aged. In L. W. Poon, ed., *Clinical memory assessment in older adults.* Washington, D.C.: American Psychological Association.

Oberleder, M. 1966. Psychotherapy with the aging: An art of the possible? *Psychotherapy: Theory, Research, and Practice* 3:139–42.

O'Conner v. *Donaldson,* 442 U.S. 563. 1975.

O'Hara, M. W., J. V. Hinrichs, F. J. Kohout, R. B. Wallace, and J. H. Lemke. 1986. Memory complaint and memory performance in depressed elderly. *Psychology and aging* 3:208–14.

Orlinsky, D. E., and K. I. Howard. 1978. The relation of process to outcome of psychotherapy. In S. L. Garfield and A. E. Bergin, eds., *Handbook of psychotherapy and behavior change.* New York: John Wiley.

Orne, M. T., and P. H. Wender. 1968. Anticipatory socialization for psychotherapy. *American Journal of Psychiatry* 124:1201–12.

Palmore, E. 1976. Total chance of institutionalization among the aged. *Gerontologist* 16:504–507.

Patterson, R. D. 1976. Services for the aged in community mental health centers. *American Journal of Psychiatry* 133:217–73.

Parsons, T. 1958. Definitions of health and illness in the light of American values and social structure. In E. Jaco, ed., *Patients, physicians and illness.* New York: Free Press.

Penner, L. A., D. A. Eberly, and R. L. Patterson. 1983. Skills training for community living. In M. A. Smyer and M. Gatz, eds., *Mental health and aging: Programs and evaluations.* Beverly Hills: Sage.

Poulschock, S. W., and G. T. Deimling. 1984. Families caring for elders in residence: Issues in measurement of burden. *Journal of Gerontology* 39:230–39.

Rabins, P., N. L. Mace, and M. J. Lucas. 1982. Impact of dementia on the family. *Journal of the American Medical Association* 248:333–35.

Rechtschaffen, A. 1959. Psychotherapy with geriatric patients. *Journal of Gerontology* 14:213–23.

Redick, R. W., and C. A. Taube. 1980. Demography and mental health care of the aged. In J. E. Birren and R. B. Sloane, eds., *Handbook of mental health and aging.* Englewood Cliffs, N. J.: Prentice Hall.

Reinhart, R. A., and S. S. Sargent. 1980. The humanistic approach: The Ventura County Creative Aging Workshops. In S. S. Sargent, ed., *Nontraditional therapy and counseling with the aging.* New York: Springer.

Robins, L. N., and Associates. 1984. Lifetime prevalence of specific psychiatric disorders in three sites. *Archives of General Psychiatry* 41:948–58.

Romanuik, M., W. J. McAuley, and G. Arling. 1983. An examination of the prevalence of mental disorders among the elderly in the community. *Journal of Abnormal Psychology* 92:458–67.

Rosecranz, H. A., and T. E. McNevin. 1969. A factor analysis of attitudes toward the aged. *Gerontologist* 9:55–59.

Rounds, J. 1982. Information and ambiguity in organizational change. In L. Sproull and P. Larkey, eds., *Advances in information processing in organizations.* Greenwich, Conn.: JAI Press.

Ruchlin, H. S., and J. N. Morris. 1983. Pennsylvania's Domiciliary Care Experiment II: Cost benefit implications. *American Journal of Public Health* 73:654–60.

Ruffin, J., and P. Urquhart. 1980. A comprehensive geriatric mental health service in San Francisco. *International Journal of Mental Health* 8:101–16.

Rypins, R. F., and M. L. Clark. 1968. A screening project for the geriatric mentally ill. *California Medicine* 109:273–78.

Sargent, S. S. 1982. Therapy and self-actualization in the late years via nontraditional approaches. *Psychotherapy: Theory, Research, and Practice* 19:522–31.

Schlossberg, N. 1984. *Counseling adults in transition.* New York: Springer.

156   *References*

Scogin, F., M. Storandt, and L. Lott. 1985. Memory skills training, memory complaints, and depression in older adults. *Journal of Gerontology* 40:562–68.
Selan, B. H., and C. A. Gold. 1980. The late life counseling services. *Hospital and Community Psychiatry* 3:403–5.
Settin, J. M. 1982. Clinical judgement in geropsychology practice. *Psychotherapy: Theory, Research, and Practice* 19:397–404.
Shadish, W. R. 1983. Comment: Costs and effects in mental health policy. *American Psychologist* 38:249–50.
Shadish, W. R. 1984. Policy research: Lessons from the implementation of deinstitutionalization. *American Psychologist* 39:725–38.
Shapiro, S., and Associates. 1984. Utilization of health and mental health services. *Archives of General Psychiatry* 41:971–78.
Sherwood, S., and J. N. Morris. 1983. The Pennsylvania Domiciliary Care Experiment I: Impact on quality of life. *American Journal of Public Health* 73:646–53.
Silverman, I. 1966. Response set bias and predictive validity associated with Kogan's "Attitudes Toward Old People Scale." *Journal of Gerontology* 21:86–88.
Spitzer, R. L., M. Gibbon, and J. Endicott. 1976. Global Assessment Scale. In A. D. Little, ed., *A working manual of sample program evaluation techniques for community mental health centers*. Department of Health, Education, and Welfare Pub. No. ADM76-404. Washington, D.C.: Government Printing Office.
Teresi, J. A., R. R. Golden, and B. J. Gurland. 1984. Concurrent and predictive validity of indicator scales developed for the comprehensive assessment and referral evaluation interview schedule. *Journal of Gerontology* 39:158–65.
Teresi, J. A., R. R. Golden, B. J. Gurland, D. E. Wilder, and R. G. Bennett. 1984. Construct validity of indicator scales developed from the comprehensive assessment and referral evaluation interview schedule. *Journal of Gerontology* 39:147–57.
Tversky, A., and D. Kahneman. 1973. Availability: A heuristic for judging frequency and probability. *Cognitive Psychology* 5:207–32.
Valle, R., and C. Martinez. 1981. Natural networks of elderly Latinos of Mexican heritage: Implications for mental health. In M. Miranda and R. A. Ruiz, eds., *Chicano aging and mental health*. Department of Health and Human Services Pub. No. ADM 81-952. Washington, D.C.: Government Printing Office.
Vanden Bos, G. R., J. Stapp, and R. Kilburg. 1981. Health service providers in psychology: Results of the APA Human Resources Survey. *American Psychologist* 36:1395–1418.
Veroff, J., P. A. Kulka, and E. Douvan. 1981. *Mental health in America*. New York: Basic Books.
Vitaliano, P. P., A. R. Breen, M. S. Albert, J. Russo, and P. N. Prinz. 1984. Memory, attention and functional status in community-residing Alzheimer-type dementia patients and optimally health age individuals. *Journal of Gerontology* 39:58–64.
Wasson, W., and Associates. 1984. Home evaluation of psychiatrically impaired elderly: Process and outcome. *Gerontologist* 24:238–41.
Wechsler, D. 1945. *Wechsler memory scale*. New York: Psychological Corporation.
Weissert, W., and W. Scanlon. November 1983. Determinants of institutionalization

of the aged. Paper presented at the meeting of the Gerontological Society of America, San Francisco.

Weissert, W., T. H. Wan, and B. B. Liveriatos. 1980. Effects and costs of day care: Homemaker services for the chronically ill. Department of Health, Education, and Welfare Pub. No. PH579-3258. Washington, D.C.: Government Printing Office.

Wollert, R. W., L. H. Levy, and B. G. Knight. 1982. Help-giving in behavioral control and stress coping self-help groups. *Small Group Behavior* 13:204–18.

Wyatt v. *Stickney*, 325 F. Supp. 781 M.D. Ala. N.C. 1971.

Zarit, S. H. 1980. *Aging and mental disorders.* New York: Free Press.

Zarit, S. H., N. Orr, and J. M. Zarit. 1985. *The hidden victims of Alzheimer's Disease.* New York: New York University Press.

Zinberg, N. E. 1964. Geriatric psychiatry: Needs and problems. *Gerontologist* 4:130–35.

Index

Vitaliano, P. P., 43
Volunteers, 13, 75

Wan, T. H., 135
Warheit, W., 133
Wasson, W., 17
Wechsler Memory Scale, 43
Weight loss, 39, 45, 46, 47
Weissert, W., 133, 135
Wender, P. H., 69, 125
Withdrawing from medical care, 15
Withdrawing from social activity, 43, 45, 46,
    57, 69

Wollert, R. W., 92
Wyatt v. *Stickney,* 12

Young adults, measuring attitudes toward the
    elderly among, 113–14
Young therapists, 55–56, 61; and effects of
    work with the elderly, 96, 101, 102

Zarit, J. M., 15, 80
Zarit, S. H., 15, 35, 42, 53, 80, 130
Zinberg, N. E., 16, 111